Solving Equine Behaviour Problems
An Equitation Science Approach

Rose M. Scofield, MRes, BSc(Hons)

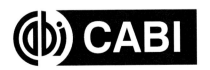

CABI is a trading name of CAB International

CABI
Nosworthy Way
Wallingford
Oxfordshire OX10 8DE
UK

Tel: +44 (0)1491 832111
Fax: +44 (0)1491 833508
E-mail: info@cabi.org
Website: www.cabi.org

CABI
WeWork
One Lincoln St
24th Floor
Boston, MA 02111
USA

Tel: +1 (617)682-9015
E-mail: cabi-nao@cabi.org

© Rose Scofield 2020. All rights reserved. No part of this publication may be reproduced in any form or by any means, electronically, mechanically, by photocopying, recording or otherwise, without the prior permission of the copyright owners.

A catalogue record for this book is available from the British Library, London, UK.

References to Internet websites (URLs) were accurate at the time of writing.

Library of Congress Cataloging-in-Publication Data

Names: Scofield, Rose, author.
Title: Solving equine behaviour problems : an equitation science approach /
    Rose M. Scofield, ResM, BSc(Hons).
Description: Wallingford, Oxfordshire ; Boston, MA : CAB International,
    [2020] | Includes bibliographical references and index. | Summary:
    "Riders can face a range of horse behavioural problems, which if left
    untreated could cause the horse-human relationship to break down. This
    book examines behavioural issues using academic research, offering
    practical solutions illustrated with photos and case studies. It covers
    over 30 major issues, including biting, kicking, shying and bolting"--Provided by publisher.
Identifiers: LCCN 2020023627 (print) | LCCN 2020023628 (ebook) | ISBN
    9781789244878 (paperback) | ISBN 9781789244885 (ebook) | ISBN
    9781789244892 (epub)
Subjects: LCSH: Horses--Behavior--Case studies. | Horses--Psychology.
Classification: LCC SF281 .S37 2020 (print) | LCC SF281 (ebook) | DDC
    636.1/0835--dc23

LC record available at https://lccn.loc.gov/2020023627
LC ebook record available at https://lccn.loc.gov/2020023628

ISBN-13: 9781789244878 (paperback)
        9781789244885 (ePDF)
        9781789244892 (ePub)

Commissioning Editor: Alexandra Lainsbury
Editorial Assistant: Lauren Davies
Production Editor: Shankari Wilford

Typeset by SPi, Pondicherry, India
Printed and bound in the UK by Severn, Gloucester

Contents

Acknowledgements

I would like to credit my students at Oxford Brookes University and Abingdon and Witney College in preparing photographs and giving up their time to be photographed. I would also like to thank my friends Chloe, Annaliese and Amber for helping me with photographs and ideas. A great debt of gratitude to my husband Simon for the diagrams and sketches.

And last but certainly not least – to all the horses I have known and loved but especially Bees, Merryn, Devon, Soda, Perry, Frank, Snopples, Teabag, Pashka, Chance and Tilly.

1 A Guide to Equitation Science

Introduction

Equitation science can be best described as a scientific explanation of the assessment of welfare while training horses, whether this takes place mounted or on the ground. This requires the appropriate evaluation of communication between human and horse, and the accurate understanding of it. The two species have great differences, though over a period of approximately 5000 years of domestication we humans would like to think the gap between us has been bridged somewhat. However, the history of horse training and therefore communication has taken a rather circuitous route, but many believe we are now at the clearest stage of this communication in our combined histories. Once a small step had been taken into the investigation of equitation science, it was clear there is much still to discover and indeed perhaps discard concerning the methods we use to communicate and therefore train our horses.

This book seeks to inform students, horse owners and caregivers about the methods of equitation science, drawing on the topic of learning theory and its basis in researched science. These discoveries about how horses learn, and therefore how we can best train them, provide the basis for solving the many behavioural problems that these intelligent animals (Fig. 1.1) can develop over their lives.

Evolution of the Horse

The earliest ancestor of the horse we know today was named 'dawn horse', or in Latin *Eohippus*, indicating the origin of all equines to be in this forest-dwelling mammal approximately the size of a medium dog. This is often disputed, and additions and subtractions made to the taxa are frequently published (McFadden, 2005). Its evolutionary history therefore is diverse and is frequently used in models to illustrate long-term aspects of evolution. Due

to this use, many textbooks include the common four-stage evolution showing its changes from a four-toed smaller mammal to a single-hoofed ungulate living in herds on the plains of America and Europe (Froehlich, 2002). However, the history of *Equus ferus caballus* is much more complicated (Fig. 1.2), although we can deduce how the horse that we know today developed its characteristics.

For all these diversifications, only one lineage survived to give rise to the horses, donkeys and zebras known today, which originated around 4–4.5 million years ago (Orlando *et al.*, 2013). The numbers of equids in these populations altered many times due to climate change, although it is thought that the Przewalski's horse and what were to become domestic horses diverged around 38,000–72,000 years ago. Indeed, Orlando *et al.* (2013) found no new admixture from the Przewalski in any of these domestic horses, demonstrating that this primitive equid does indeed embody the only existing genetic example of wild horses (Fig. 1.3). However, it appears that the Przewalski's horses living today have all been bred from captive individuals, demonstrating that there are no genuine wild horses left (Lau *et al.*, 2009).

It is important to consider this lineage in the domestication of the horse, because of the common thread throughout their history, indicating the adaptation of this forest-dwelling mammal to a fast-paced, long-legged mammal with fixed vertebrae, a very convoluted digestive system and complicated communication system. Equine communication incorporates a whole plethora of body signals, eye movements, vocalization and pheromone release, making it rather easy for humans to misinterpret exactly what their horses are communicating. The domestication of the horse by humans around 5500 years ago impacted positively on physiological traits such as limb strength, cardiac refinement and musculature (Schubert *et al.*, 2014). Interestingly, psychological traits including learning ability, response to fearful situations and

© R. Scofield 2020. *Solving Equine Behaviour Problems* (R. Scofield)

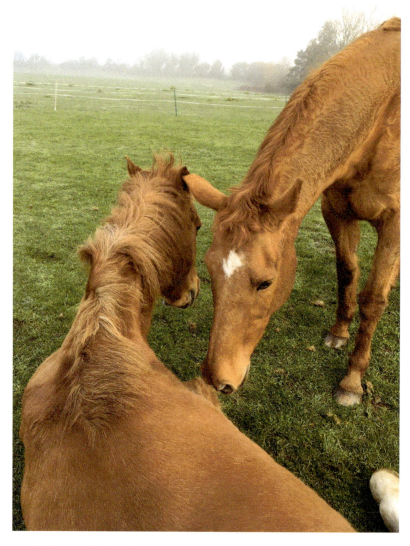

Fig. 1.1. Horses are intelligent animals and companionship is of great importance to them.

social behaviour were also impacted favourably, suggesting humans involved with the domestication of horses were indeed selecting for temperament.

While domestication has given the horse longevity in the provision of medical care, husbandry and usefulness this has not necessarily been in line with its evolutionary behavioural requirements (Goodwin, 1999). Horses evolved to run, to live in herds, and to communicate with each other in a rich and varied way and these behavioural needs cannot be truly satisfied in a domestic setting. Today, the problems of undesirable behaviour almost certainly stem from a misunderstanding of the horse's needs, and in the necessity of humans to keep horses how we want them to be, rather than what they evolved for (Fig. 1.4). A row of stables in a barn, while being very practical for humans, may deny the occupants chances to communicate through touch (Fig. 1.5). It will restrict their movement, their choice of foodstuffs, and their innate desire to breed. Even horses living out at pasture all their lives will not have the choice of natural groupings, or large living spaces, and all will probably at some time be ridden or used in other ways, such as driving.

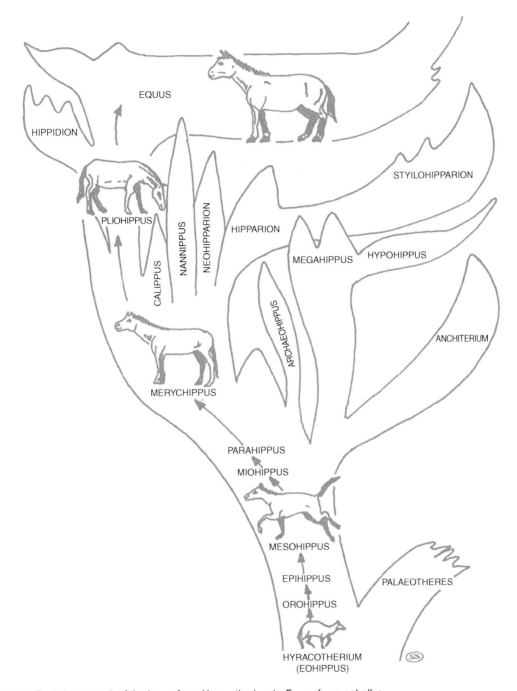

Fig. 1.2. Evolutionary path of the horse from *Hyracotherium* to *Equus ferus caballus*.

Behavioural problems do arise from many different sources, some of which are never discovered and remain a mystery. The use of ethology combined with knowledge of the evolutionary background of the horse can help to solve these issues, and an informed understanding of learning theory is vital for any retraining that may be needed.

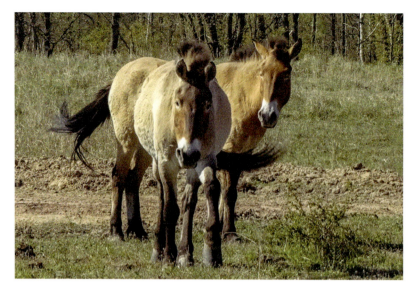

Fig. 1.3. English feral Przewalski horses at nature reserve. (Döberitzer Heide)

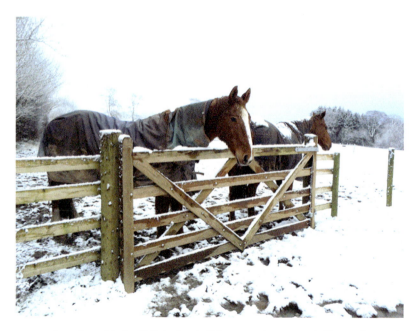

Fig. 1.4. Horses cope extremely well in the British climate if they are given enough fibre and rugged well.

Stabling, Turnout and its Effects on Behaviour

Horses in the UK are kept in a variety of systems: those known as 'living-out', where horses have no time in a stable; a combination system, where they have access to pasture but spend part of the day or night inside; or stabled, where they spend all their time inside and do not have access to pasture. The different systems have some relation to the use of the horse and the disciplines it takes part in, but there are crossovers in all cases. For example,

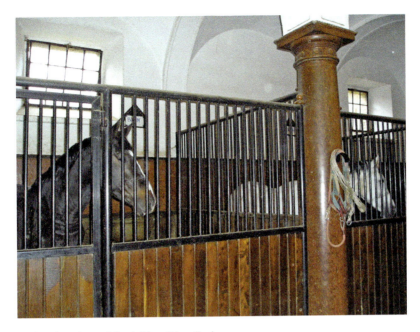

Fig. 1.5. Horses in American barn style stables. (Magellan)

all race and competition horses are usually in a combination system or are stabled, but polo ponies tend to live out (Fig. 1.6). Most leisure horses are either in a combination system or live out, but there are yards that do keep them stabled, particularly if pasture is at a premium or the weather has been inclement. Many racehorses have limited access to pasture when they are in training but tend to live out when they are in their rest period or are in rehabilitation. Dressage and show jumping horses often spend much of their time stabled.

There are many reasons for the use of different systems, and for many owners and riders the reasons for keeping horses on a combination or stabled system tend to be to do with the weather and/ or pasture availability (Fig. 1.7). If riders have limited amounts of time in their day to exercise horses, keeping them in may be the only option to avoid spending precious time grooming muddy coats. Another consideration is flies and biting insects: horses are much more likely to be irritated by these if they live out, and those with medical conditions such as sweet itch (a reaction to a type of midge bite) may need to be in when the insects are active (Fig. 1.9). Weather is of course not just mud – a very hot summer can also affect some horses and may result in sunburnt muzzles in pale or grey horses that have connections to ill health.

However, there are now emerging motives for horses to have as much turnout as is possible and some of these are discussed below.

Stabling versus turnout

The study of behaviour in all the different systems of keeping horses has produced some interesting research, much of which does indicate that giving horses as much turnout in an outside area, such as a paddock, as is possible is most beneficial (Fig. 1.8). When desirable and undesirable behaviours were studied, more of those described as desirable were observed in horses that were turned out (Losonci and Paddison, 2016). It was also reported that those horses turned out were easier to handle, even when compared with animals stabled for only one day. It appears, therefore, that the effect of being stabled for even short periods impacts on horses in an adverse way. Physical findings corroborate these behavioural observations, and horses that were stabled showed abnormality in blood cell count that did not return to normal even if they had time out in paddocks during the day (Le Simple et al., 2020). Their behavioural repertoires were also enhanced, however, with stereotypical actions declining if they had experienced turnout (Fig. 1.10). The effects noticed in this study were directly related to the turnout

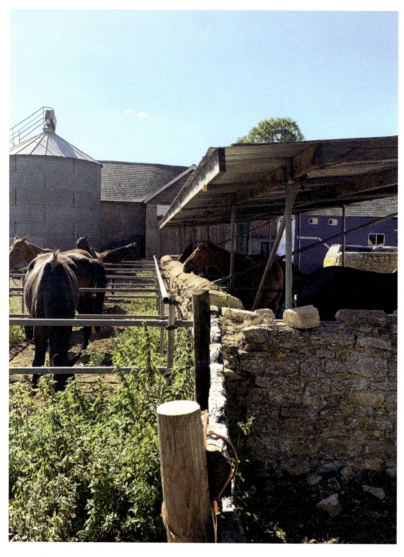

Fig. 1.6. Polo pony stalls showing the ability of the horses to communicate with each other.

periods, as when they were stabled again the indicators quickly reverted to earlier levels, demonstrating lower welfare when stabled. Indeed, when compared with hacking horses in stable social groups that lived out, horses in riding school conditions (stabled, with reduced access to fibre and ridden by novice riders) displayed much higher levels of behavioural problems (Henry *et al.*, 2017). The riding school horses also had raised levels of illness and what was described as a less 'positive' outlook.

Another effect that stabling appears to have with horses is related to training and 'willingness' or ability to learn. Quite a number of studies have uncovered data suggesting that those horses kept on pasture have higher rates of learning capability, including the capacity of adaptation to training shown by those horses experiencing turnout (Rivera *et al.*, 2002). Willingness to perform has unknown qualities, with many owners anecdotally describing their horses as 'willing' or 'uncooperative', when it is not sure scientifically what is meant by this, other than a possible reaction to motivation. However, horsepersons are comfortable with the description, and this willingness has been reported as slightly higher in

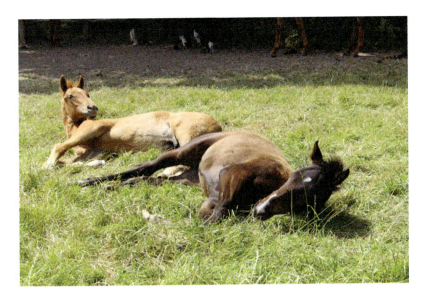

Fig. 1.7. Foals relaxing in a summer field.

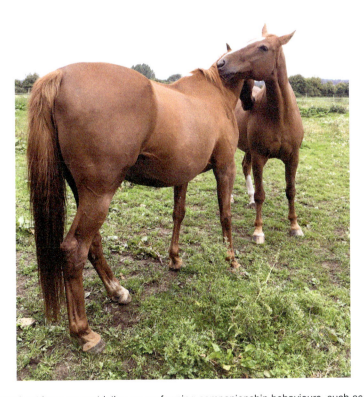

Fig. 1.8. Horses turned out have no restriction on performing companionship behaviours, such as these two horses displaying the common behaviour of mutual grooming, known as allogrooming.

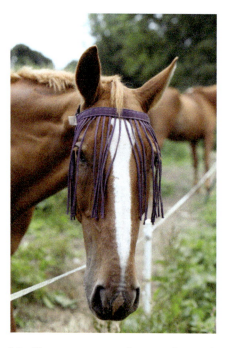

Fig. 1.9. Flies can prove a nuisance to horses that live out, but can be managed with simple fly fringes or fly masks.

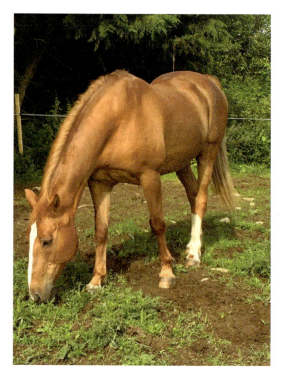

Fig. 1.10. A horse turned out in the spring. Grass is rapidly covering muddy areas left from the winter.

horses that are completely field kept (Werhahn *et al.*, 2012). If a horse is under stress of some kind, perhaps due to lack of companionship or access to food, which can happen as part of a stabled horse's life, this can impact on the ability to train, and indeed stress levels were seen as elevated in horses with no turnout at all (Werhahn *et al.*, 2012). Due to these findings, it is worth considering extra turnout for all horses to improve their welfare even if it is at the expense of the humans looking after them (Fig. 1.10).

The use of enrichment in stables

When considering improvements in all the areas concerned with the stabling of horses, parallels with risk factors involving hacking horses and competition horses appeared to be very similar (Hockenhull and Creighton, 2014). It seems that there is no difference in risk factors across all types of horse use when they are stabled, and what is characteristic and appropriate for performance horses does not change when applied to hacking horses. There is a large body of evidence and experiment concerning stereotypies, a concern for all horse owners, due to the physical and mental effects they cause. There

seems to be no difference between hacking and performance horses – though those with less access to hay and/or haylage and companionship (which may point to turnout) perhaps develop stereotypies more often than field-kept animals.

Consequently, horsepersons trial different methods to stop or alleviate stereotypies and one of these is the use of mirrors in stables. There is evidence to suggest that providing a mirror in the stable does reduce the incidence of the stereotypy of weaving (McAfee *et al.*, 2002), and this decrease continued for a 5-week period. There are reports that the use of a mirror does decline after time but may well prove useful for a while. Other objects include those containing appetitive 'licks', balls on ropes and also a 'feed-ball', where a portion of the horse's mix is put into a ball that rolls around the stable when touched and dispenses food. There are issues particularly with the feed-ball, where it is very beneficial for predatory animals such as cats and dogs (Heath and Wilson, 2014) but perhaps misaligned with horses, who are grazing prey animals with no need to hunt in a similar way. However, the only research to date with feed-balls in stabled horses did report a decrease in stereotypical behaviours (Henderson and Waran, 2001), so their use should be considered in these cases.

Other research investigating the addition of parameters to aid the welfare of stabled horses has considered the application of music to the environment. 'New Age' relaxing music appeared to lower the heart rate of geriatric horses in stabled conditions, but the effect only lasted for 2 weeks, reducing significantly after this time (Wisniewska *et al.*, 2019). However, when an experiment used composed music with Arabian racehorses, the effect appeared to be sustained for up to 3 months, reducing heart rate considerably in this time and also having an effect on performance and prize-winning (Stachurska *et al.*, 2015). For horses in stressful situations, such as transport in this experiment, the use of classical music displayed a quicker post-stress recovery of heart rate when used in a sample of animals (Neveux *et al.*, 2016). The addition of music has also been reported to have a significantly positive effect on sleeping horses, increasing their time in sleep when stabled to closer mimic that of field-kept horses (Hartman and Greening, 2019). Music does appear to have a beneficial effect on horse welfare, though reports do differ on the length of time that it is advantageous. However, there does appear to be consensus that the category of music should be either classical or relaxing, and perhaps the common sight of a radio hung up playing in many stables should be selected to a classical music station in the future.

Bedding – the advantages of straw

Many experiments have considered straw bedding, and its comparison with other types used in stables for horses on combination systems and those stabled for 24 hours a day. Straw bedding is frequently used in the UK, being generally cheaper than other kinds such as shavings, elephant grass and wood pellets, but reported anecdotally as being heavier to work with and not so absorbent. Many livery yards have restrictions on the form of bedding allowed, with preference for those that rot down more easily or that contractors will remove. Each owner or stable worker, if asked, would prefer a certain type of bedding, and this may be related to quickness of mucking out, smell, ability to handle the product, plus the issues of horses eating certain sorts. Another issue with bedding is related to its degree of dust or particulates that are shed as it is worked and used by the horse. Dusty bedding material sometimes contains a fungus identified as *Aspergillus fumigatus* on the particles, giving rise to a condition called recurrent airway obstruction (commonly known as chronic obstructive pulmonary disorder, or 'heaves'), which can ultimately lead to breathlessness and necessary euthanasia if not managed correctly. Straw contains less particulates than other bedding (Nazarenko *et al.*, 2018), so it may be a natural choice for prevention and management. Also, horses certainly perform less stereotypies if bedded on straw, due to the availability of the straw to graze on once their hay ration has been eaten; however, this is not necessarily a good enough reason for horsepersons to change to straw use.

Nevertheless, behavioural repertoires are affected if straw is used, with relaxation increased and playing with bedding occurring, whereas other types tend to promote aggressive behaviours and pacing (Kwiatkowska-Stenzel *et al.*, 2016). These include biting, and threatening to bite horses stabled next to them, and locomotory behaviours such as box-walking. When compared with shavings and wood pellet bedding, straw again proved the most desirable, with enhanced encouraging behavioural ranges amongst the horses tested (Werhahn *et al.*, 2010). Straw therefore appears to enhance desirable behavioral repertoires, proving an improved environment for stabled horses, which is undoubtedly beneficial, particularly if they do not have access to pasture.

Other issues with bedding and owner preference relate to the use of 'banks', or piling bedding up at the walls of the box, thought to protect horses from injuring themselves when getting up and down. Currently no research has studied the use of banks, but there may be issues in the reduction of space in the stable with large banks, and indeed they may prove only to be for the benefit of the owner who thinks they are visually more attractive. The thickness of beds is also a consideration: horses do tend to stand less if the bedding is placed thickly on the floor (Guay *et al.*, 2019), hence it is recommended to bed horses as densely as possible (Fig. 1.11). Another related technique is known as 'deep litter', where bedding is left down every day, with wet patches of urine and faeces removed and a new layer of bedding put on top. This system can be used for as long as is required but cleaning it out will get more difficult as it gets older, wetter and heavier. Mucking out and the movement of bedding in the stable area, and particularly in the American barn system where horses live in separate stables enclosed in a

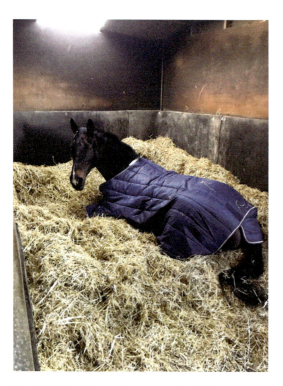

Fig. 1.11. Bedding such as straw placed thickly on the stable floor is preferred by horses.

building, causes high levels of particulates (Claussen and Hessel, 2017), so a deep-litter system may be recommended to reduce the possibility of development of ill health. However, the issue of best practice in deep-litter systems must also be explored, because if not sufficiently removed faeces and wet patches could contribute to a hostile environment for horses' hooves and thus promote thrush or other conditions seen in these circumstances.

Feeding fibre

Fibre or roughage provision for horses has always been a talking point for owners and handlers, with not just the different types and their nutritional content, but also how they are fed. Traditionally, horses in stables had head-height metal racks, into which hay was thrown from a barn or store above. After these storage facilities disappeared, the metal racks were still used, until with progress came the hay net available in all different sizes and colours. Hay nets are generally tied up on a ring with the use of thinner and weaker baler twine as an intermediary, in case the horse gets a foot caught in the net and needs to break away from it. The height of

hay nets has long been debated, and certainly many horse owners now feed from the ground, or some sort of hay-feeder in the corner of the stable. Unfortunately, this method does tend to waste the expensive fibre, so there is ultimately a discussion to be had around which is preferable. It is surmised that feeding hay from any sort of height reduces the ability of the mucus to clear particulates from the trachea, as it is not draining naturally downwards, and this is often given as a reason for the floor method to be used.

Using hay nets has also been reported to increase frustration for horses, perhaps due to the extra foraging that is needed to pull hay through the holes in the netting. Medium- and small-holed hay nets did indeed increase the performance of frustration behaviours in horses when compared with large-hole nets (Glunk *et al.*, 2014). The relatively modern invention known as a 'hay-bag', where hay is delivered to the horse in a large bag made from durable fabric instead of a netted material, has also been reported to cause these frustration behaviours (Rochais *et al.*, 2018). In the same study, horses eating from 'slow-feeders', those positioned on the floor with easier access for horses to eat from, had a reduced level of stereotypies, and there was even a noticeable difference in their responsiveness towards humans. However, hay nets with small holes do decrease eating times by as much as 5 minutes per kilogram of fibre (Ellis *et al.*, 2015), and also tend to extend eating time throughout the night. Another observation was slightly concerning, in that by half-past ten at night a significant number of the subjects had finished their available ration, leaving a lengthy time before those horses were fed again.

The provision of fibre is serious and many factors need to be considered. The time budgets of feral horses involve 14–22 hours of feeding every day. The lack of ability to mimic this natural behaviour in a stabled environment is worrying, and indeed has involved many studies regarding the development of ulcers in horses not fed enough fibre. Conversely, there is the all too real problem of overfeeding and obesity in horses, certainly a reason why owners may want to restrict their horse's intake. Each owner must decide how their horse will be fed, but should perhaps base their decisions on science rather than tradition.

Aspects concerning horses that live out in groups

Horses that have access to 24-hour turnout may live in groups of varying sizes and incorporating different ages, sexes and breeds. Many livery yards and owners tend to split horses into grazing groups that they think might reduce injury, such as the common method of keeping mares and geldings separately, or youngsters separate from veteran horses. Conventional methods of horses being separated into males and females are commonplace, and seen amongst not just leisure horses but also sports and performance animals. Nevertheless, there seems to be no scientific evidence that these methods work to prevent problems, as disparities in ages and sexes had negligible effect on injury quantities (Fig. 1.12), handling and, even more important when considering behaviour, the reactivity of the horses (Keeling *et al.*, 2016).

However, these social groups need careful management, as changes in their make-up can affect the dynamics of the horses involved (Fig. 1.13). If a horse needs to be taken out of the group, there may be issues of separation anxiety, therefore the group is better kept smaller and managed between owners. Regular changes to groups of horses do not appear to have encouraging effects on the relationships between the individuals (Christensen *et al.*, 2011a) so keeping numbers as stable as possible is recommended. It is known that horses do not have any hierarchy as such, and it is certainly not helpful for humans to try to assume leadership roles in social groups of horses where they probably do not exist (Hartmann *et al.*, 2017). Consequently, when taking horses out of groups for riding or other reasons, handlers must practice safe behaviour and be aware of the characteristics of each herd member.

Understanding Learning Theory

Since the beginnings of domestication, methods of horse training have evolved with the support of experience passed down from teacher to student in the passage of time. The advent of equitation science, with its body of researchers drawn from all the multi-factorial fields of the study of the horse, has given access to a plethora of published studies. These have influenced equine regulations and laws around the world, including the whip rules in racing and the emergence of noseband tightness measuring in some European countries.

In the late 19th and early 20th centuries, scientists such as Ivan Pavlov and Burrhus Frederic (B.F.) Skinner carried out experiments in learning ability. After the middle of the 20th century a new science called

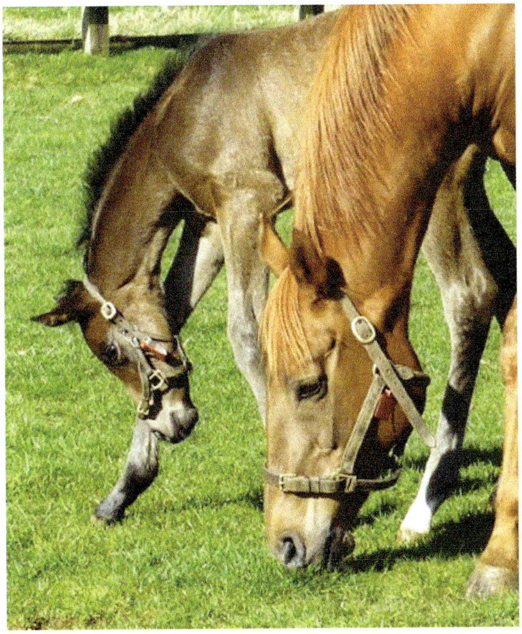

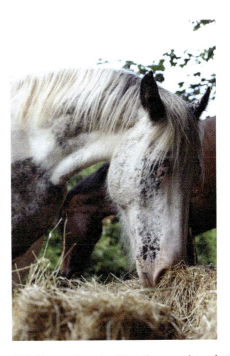

Fig. 1.12. A mix of ages does not appear to affect rates of injury in groups of horses kept out together.

Fig. 1.13. Horses turned out together must have free access to fibre if needed, and to avoid injury each animal needs to be able to reach the source without bickering amongst the group.

ethology began to add to the interpretation of animal learning: it investigated natural behaviour and how animals learn from their parents or which innate abilities they are born with. The scientific theory of learning was therefore established and studied in many varieties of animals, thus forming a body of evidence for the study of training in many animals.

Associative learning

Classical conditioning

Pavlov, a name known to many for his research on dogs, was the first to publish extensively about how animals will learn to respond to an unconnected event if that event occurs before some sort of reward (Pavlov, 1927). His experiments on the digestive systems of dogs suggested a connection between their salivation episodes and the appearance of the assistant who fed them. Pavlov introduced a metronome sound (often illustrated as a bell) before they were fed and discovered that the dogs would salivate on the sound of the device, before the food even appeared. The concept is based on conditioning the animal to a stimulus that has no actual connection with the reward, so the noise is played before the

food is delivered, and the animal quickly connects the stimulus of the food with the stimulus of the noise and salivates even when only the noise is heard, because it has been conditioned to expect the food (Fig. 1.14). Today, this method of training is named classical conditioning, and is used in many different scenarios in the training or retraining of horses, and sometimes as a response to the environment not even realized.

An example of classical conditioning in horse training occurs in foundation training (the first training a horse receives to ready it for a rider) when inadvertently horses will learn to respond to a clicking noise made by its rider and speed up its pace. The rider may be giving the signal to move forward, that is pressure from their lower leg against the flank, and at the same time unconsciously make the familiar clicking noise. The horse responds to this as a stimulus for moving forward and then the rider may find that clicking alone will make the horse react. If trainers understand classical conditioning, they can add this to their techniques and use it in many varying circumstances; for example, shaking a bucket and calling a horse in from the field – they will even find the rattling of the bucket is enough of a stimulus to provoke a response.

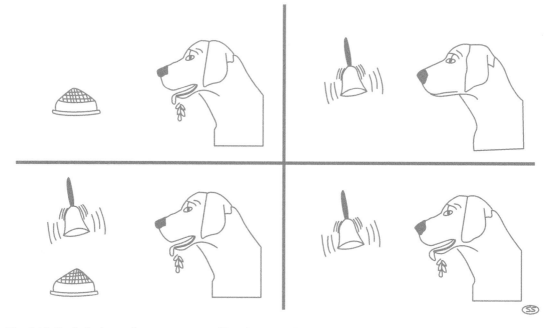

Fig. 1.14. Pavlov's dogs – the consequence of learning a conditioned response (salivation) to a conditioned stimulus (the bell) without the presence of the original unconditioned stimulus (food).

Operant conditioning

Also known as trial and error learning, the mechanism of operant conditioning involves a reward for effort, and was first investigated by Edward Thorndike in his Law of Effect, where the addition of a pleasant consequence after an action seems to initiate a repeat of the action and where the addition of punishment appears to reduce a repeat of the action (Thorndike, 1898). Thorndike discovered that when a cat in a holding box was exposed to a lever, and could see or smell food, it would use trial and error to try to reach the food. Eventually it might step on the lever, releasing the trapdoor and allowing access to food (Fig. 1.15). The cat would then be placed back inside the box and allowed to trial behaviours again until the lever was pressed, and the food made available. After a few trials the cat began to learn that if it pressed the lever the trapdoor would open, and from that moment the cat would immediately press the lever on entry into the box. Latency (time taken) to learn procedures such as these and become conditioned to responding to gain the reward varies across species, and with horses varies greatly (Craig *et al.*, 2015).

Skinner developed the idea of operant conditioning further, basing his studies on Thorndike's research with cats but instead using rats and pigeons. He demonstrated that by using repetition the individual animal learns that a particular action brings a pleasant consequence and therefore it tends to be repeated by the animal (Skinner, 1938). He demonstrated that where a behaviour or action is repeated using operant conditioning it is reinforced and is more likely to be repeated and then strengthens in its potency. Operant conditioning used in this way for training with horses can be described as either positive reinforcement or negative reinforcement, and the student of learning theory must remember that in this context positive means 'addition' of an appetitive reward, and negative refers to a 'subtraction' of an aversive stimulus, thus providing the reward in its removal. Negative does not mean that it is an aversive method of training, rather that it uses the removal of an aversive stimulus as the reward the animal works for. Due to confusion in the understanding behind the terms of positive and negative, it has been suggested they should be renamed as 'addition reinforcement' and 'subtraction reinforcement' in an endeavour to clarify their true meaning (McGreevy *et al.*, 2017).

The theory of using a positive (addition), or appetitive, stimulus also came from Skinner's research. He demonstrated with hungry rats activating a lever in his Skinner Box by accident and causing a food reward to appear. In a short period of time the rats learnt that the consequence of activating the lever was crucial to obtaining the food reward, and then displayed this learnt behaviour repeatedly when put in the box (Fig. 1.16). If this experiment was repeated, or reinforced, the behaviour became learnt.

Conversely, the use of negative (subtraction) reinforcement involves the removal of an unpleasant stimulus, which also acts as a reward because it stops the unpleasant experience. The animal therefore learns that if an unpleasant stimulus is applied, and it stops

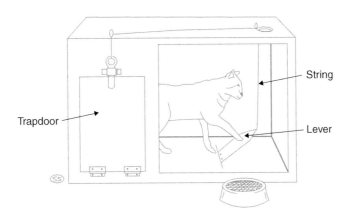

Fig. 1.15. Thorndike's cats – pressing on the lever releases the trapdoor so the cat can reach the food. By trial and error the cat learns to press the lever and open the door.

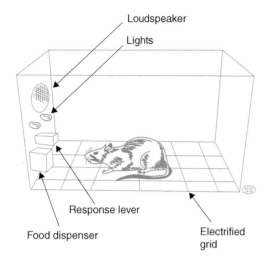

Loudspeaker

Lights

Response lever

Food dispenser

Electrified grid

Fig. 1.16. Skinners Box – the rat is placed on an electrified grid with a lever which the rat can press to release food, and also to stop any electric shock. It quickly learns to press the lever when the light turns on to warn it of the impending shock.

its present action, it is rewarded by the cessation of the stimulus. This action is also strengthened by repetition. Skinner exhibited this by using an electric shock stimulus that was stopped when a rat knocked the lever. As with the positive reinforcement experiment, the rat soon learnt to operate the lever in order to stop the shock. The consequence again showed that the rats would repeat the process on learning the sequence of events. Skinner developed this further by using a light source before the electric shock started, and maybe as expected the rats learnt to operate the lever because they had learnt it would halt the use of the electric stimulus.

Positive and negative reinforcement examples in horses

An example of negative reinforcement in horse training might be the use of what is also known as 'pressure-release', sometimes used as a descriptor for negative reinforcement in horses as this is how it is commonly used. When training a horse to move forward, pressure is applied to the flanks and then removed when the horse begins to walk. The aversive stimulus is the pressure, and the learnt behaviour of walking forward is reinforced by the removal of this pressure as the reward. Most training with horses uses this concept, such as stopping a horse with pressure on a bit or a bitless bridle noseband, asking a horse

to move forwards or backwards with pressure on the lead rope. Horses readily learn with negative reinforcement, possibly due to their use of pressure in communication with other horses (Fig. 1.17) and it seems in some cases also with humans. For this reason, negative reinforcement is in use by every ridden training programme, even though it is not recognized as such in many cases (Fenner *et al.*, 2017). Horses use pressure in their own conspecific relationships, so when pressure-release (as negative reinforcement) is used as a training method it is largely very successful (Ahrendt *et al.*, 2015). The act of asking a horse to move forwards is generally accomplished by pressure on the horse's flanks, which should then be removed immediately when the animal responds. Problems can develop when this aversive pressure is not removed as soon as a response is seen (Kydd *et al.*, 2017). If the pressure is not removed, there is no reward and the horse does not learn. This can develop into a condition where novice riders 'train' a horse inadvertently to lose their response either to hand on the reins/bit or to legs on the flank, creating what is termed a 'hard mouth' or a horse that is 'dead to the leg'.

Positive reinforcement proves more difficult to use in horse training, particularly when riding, as the horse needs to trial the behaviour and then be rewarded once it performs correctly – very difficult to accomplish when riding. This method of learning is possibly best used when training horses to accept aversive procedures, such as clipping or shoeing. With clipping, the horse may not be inclined to stand still, but could be asked to stand and then rewarded with a treat once it does so. In the case of positive reinforcement horses generally have a high drive towards food rewards, so their motivation to learn and complete a task is strong (Fig. 1.18). Horses can be trained to touch objects on word command using positive reinforcement with appetite reward (Ferguson and Rosales-Ruiz, 2001) and then will also generalize to other similar items.

It is therefore possible to teach horses to touch targets (Fig. 1.19) and this can prove useful in various situations, such as asking a horse to load into a trailer without the use of negative reinforcement. In trailer training for difficult loaders, positive reinforcement when trialled in comparison with negative reinforcement produced horses demonstrating fewer stressful behaviours with shorter training periods, though heart rate did not differ between the two groups (Hendriksen *et al.*, 2010). With ponies and horses in a rehabilitation programme, the group

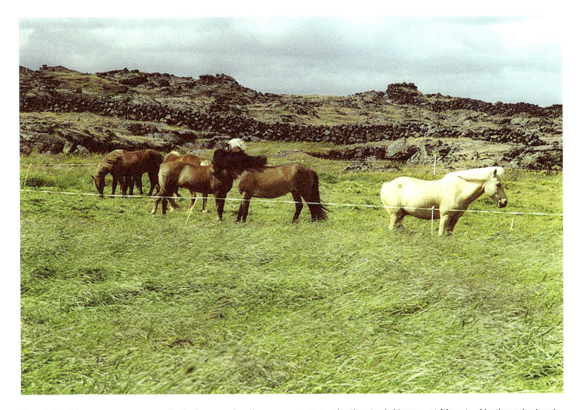

Fig. 1.17. Horses use pressure in their everyday lives as a communication tool. Horses at Myvatn, Northern Iceland. (Julius Agrippa.)

trained with positive reinforcement demonstrated more motivation in the training periods and tended to display a larger amount of investigative behaviour (Innes and McBride, 2008). The evidence tends to point towards the use of positive reinforcement if it is possible; however, as explained, this approach of reinforcement is very difficult to apply in the ridden horse.

Reinforcement in either method becomes fixed if the experiment, or training in the case of animals, is repeated. However, if the reward in both instances is eventually stopped, the behaviour will slowly become extinguished and will disappear, or become, as it is called, 'extinct'. Interestingly, if the learning process is started again, the animal will quickly remember the training, and will start to respond as it did before. In some cases, animals will unexpectedly trial the learnt behaviour in different circumstances, even if the trainer is sure it has been extinguished, and this can be problematic. An example occurred in the case of a horse taught to lift either its left or right front leg in response either to a command, or

to the signal of the owner also raising their leg on one or other side of the horse. The animal readily learnt this technique and responded very quickly to the training. However, after a while it was noticed that the horse would trial this behaviour in other circumstances, such as when waiting for food or being tacked up if it was in an arousal state. The answer was to let the behaviour naturally become extinct, by removing any type of reward or communication with the horse when it performed the pawing gesture. Eventually it did become extinct, but to this day the horse sometimes still trials the old pawing behaviour, even though it was learnt many years ago.

Schedules of reinforcement

Ferster and Skinner (1957) investigated varied ways of using operant conditioning for learning, including the response rate of rats pressing the lever, and the extinction rate or how long it took for the rats to stop pressing the lever once the reward was

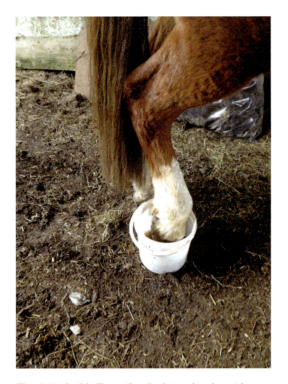

Fig. 1.18. In this illustration the horse has learnt by positive reinforcement to place its hoof in a bucket for treatment of an abscess.

removed. They discovered that rats would learn more quickly if the reward was given at erratic times, so sometimes they got the reward after operating the lever and sometimes they did not. This also lengthened time to extinction of the learnt behaviour, due to its unpredictability, and is known as variable ratio reinforcement in learning theory. In contrast, if a reward is given every time the behaviour is performed, extinction rate is faster due to the anticipation of receiving it, so when it ceases, the behaviour quickly becomes extinct. This method of reward, known as continuous reinforcement, also has a benefit to the animal involved as it reduces the stress of expectancy as experienced with variable ratio reinforcement; however, it takes longer to learn overall. The variable schedules of reinforcement all have their uses in training, and in retraining, and can be selected according to the problem behaviour experienced, its aetiology, and the characteristics of the horse displaying the problem (Fig. 1.20).

Differential reinforcement of other behaviour

A recognized technique used in humans to reduce self-harming (Cowdery *et al.*, 1990), this method has also been investigated in horse training (Fox *et al.*, 2012). It involves a reward being offered when the

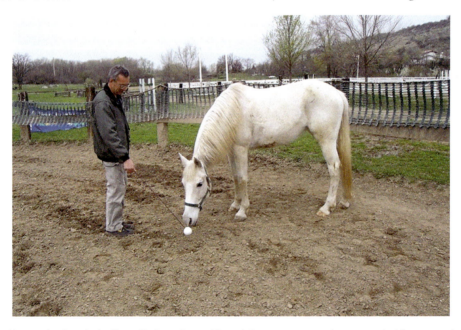

Fig. 1.19. Horses (and ponies) will readily learn by positive reinforcement to touch a target, in this case a simple stick. (Brollo, 2006.)

Chapter 1

Method of reinforcement	Fixed-ratio	Variable-ratio	Fixed-interval schedule	Variable-interval schedule
When reward is given	After a specified number of responses	After an unpredictable number of responses	After a specified amount of time	After an unpredictable amount of time
Response to stimulus	High steady rate of response	High steady rate of response	High response near the end of the interval, slower immediately afterwards	Slow steady rate of response

Fig. 1.20. Schedules of reinforcement.

horse is not performing the undesirable behaviour, so it is described as a reversal design rather than the reward being dependent on performing a behaviour. For example, if a horse is reluctant to stand and keeps moving about, it is only rewarded when it is still and has stopped any locomotion. This acts to lessen the undesirable behaviour, as the horse then learns that standing still is the behaviour that is rewarded and moving around is not worth the expenditure as there is no reward to fuel its motivation (Fig. 1.21). It is an interesting concept that has proven very useful in the retraining of problems in horses and is described in some case studies in the following chapters for this purpose.

One-trial learning

The evolution of the horse has a large part to play in the way it learns, and none more so than the phenomenon of one-trial learning. As prey animals, horses would need to learn extremely quickly that a certain shape and movement (such as a stalking predator) meant danger, and the ability to react quickly to this certain shape would ensure survival. Therefore, horses can learn to react to fearful situations in one trial, or one experience, and once learned these behaviours can become almost inextinguishable (LeDoux, 1994). Horses will tend to revert to these 'hard-wired' learnt behaviours in stressful situations (Grandin and Deesing, 2014), often not related at all to the original incident, but used as the 'go-to' response. For example, a frightened horse that reacts with a rearing action may

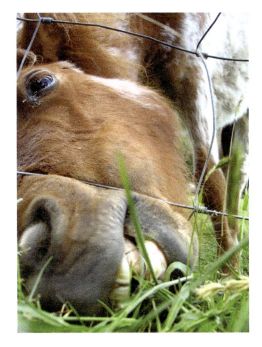

Fig. 1.21. Reward for the horse can take any form – it is useful to discover what reward motivates your horse the most. (Frenkieb from Netherlands.)

have learnt that this stopped the incessant kicking or whipping from the rider when they tried to force the animal to move forward into what it perceived as a dangerous area. Such responses as rearing can therefore become fixed and trialled again in very different stressful situations, such as loading into a trailer or show jumping. In training, humans must be very wary of this learning process, as it can be the instigator of many undesirable behavioural problems.

Successive approximation (shaping)

Skinner identified that when using operant conditioning, with either positive or negative reinforcement, animal learning can be aided by an idea he named 'successive approximation' (Skinner, 1951). This is identified as rewarding an animal for a near attempt at performing the wanted behaviour; for instance, the rat in question would receive a reward for moving near the lever or touching it even though it did not actually operate it. In this way, the behaviour is shaped and reinforced so that it is more likely to happen correctly on the next try, with further modifications by the animal leading to the completion of the task. Shaping is extremely useful to the behaviourist who is attempting to retrain a problem behaviour in a horse. It enables early reward to be given to the horse, which encourages it and motivates it to perform the wanted behaviour. For example, in the case of target training for ease of loading into a trailer the horse can be rewarded if it merely moves its muzzle towards the target, and this will act to encourage it to trial the behaviour again as its motivation is naturally higher. Every circumstance where reinforcement is used can first be shaped to encourage the horse towards correctly completing the task.

Punishment

The use of punishment in animal training and particularly dog training, once popular, is slowly being eradicated due to the detrimental effects on the welfare of the animal involved (Shalvey et al., 2019). This form of training is, however, still very current in horse training, with use of the whip or crop when a horse does not attempt a jump, or a smack from a hand on the muzzle when they bite. This abuse is seen on a regular basis from people handling horses in every discipline from 'happy hackers' or leisure horses to performance animals. When used as part of a horse's regular training, there is a significant rise in the number of problem behaviours reported (Padalino et al., 2018). Apart from the ethical issues raised when abusing animals by hitting them, there are various reasons that should mean the elimination of punishment in

horses by handlers and riders even if the increase of their horse's welfare is not of concern to them.

Effects of punishment on horses were first documented in the mid-1980s (Voith, 1986), and consist of several reactions that occur when it is used as a training method. The first appears to be an increase of aggressive behaviours from the horse towards the person hitting it (Mills, 1998), without an understanding of why it is being hit in the first instance. For example, a horse may unintentionally step on a person's foot, and the person hits it. The horse will fail to understand what this means, but it will attach the pain and aggression to the human involved, and this may make the horse more fearful of them. Fear itself is increased with punishment, and the generation of fear may manifest in undesirable behaviours (Bradshaw, 2009). A fearful aggressive horse will not be a pleasant animal to have contact with, especially if it also needs to be trained and ridden by the person delivering the punishment.

Apart from creating a more aggressive and fearful horse, regular punishment also acts as a limiting action on the ability to learn (Parker et al., 2008). It tends to suppress the unwanted behaviour until the punishment stops, not actually extinguish it like reinforcement is proven to do. Additionally, the use of punishment is also counter-indicative in training, as it does not teach the animal what to do, but rather what not to do (Mills, 1998). Punishment is therefore a direct opposite to reinforcement, where it attempts to weaken the unwanted behaviour rather than reinforcing the correct one. Horsepersons must be proactive and make sure that they understand the pitfalls of punishment if they want to include it in their training programmes. Also, it is very important for anyone dealing with horses that they understand the difference between punishment and negative reinforcement. When negative reinforcement is used in training there must be absolute attention to the removal of the aversive stimulus, for reward to take place. If this is not done, such as the pressure on a rein is not released quickly enough once the horse responds, it can metamorphose into punishment with all the impact on welfare that this method of training brings.

Non-associative learning
Habituation

Learning theory incorporates habituation as a method of training without using operant conditioning, so

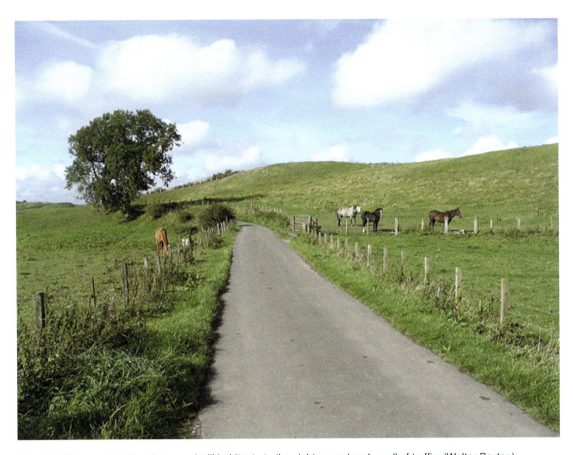

Fig. 1.22. Horses turned out by a road will habituate to the sight, sound and smell of traffic. (Walter Baxter.)

the animal learns itself that a situation, change or addition to its environment stops being frightening and, due to familiarity, is not worth reacting to (Christensen, 2013). For instance, a horse that is easily scared by traffic could certainly be less so if it is kept in a pasture with a busy road next to it (Fig. 1.22). The horse soon learns that even though the continuous vehicles may at first be aversive, they do not impact directly on the animal and it is not worth expending energy by running away from the noise/movement. The once-frightening stimulus therefore becomes less so when the animal has a continuous experience of it and learns it is not worth reacting to. This can prove stressful, as the situation or change that the animal is subjected to can be very frightening at first and can raise stress levels higher than the method of desensitization (Fureix *et al.*, 2009a). An example of this procedure used in humans is exposure therapy (or 'flooding'), where the subject

is exposed to whatever is aversive to it with no steps to reach this full experience.

Systematic desensitization

The method of desensitization is often confused with habituation, where an animal is exposed immediately to the threatening situation. Desensitization involves stages of exposure to a novel or frightening object, or a fear hierarchy, so that the animal slowly becomes accustomed to it over a period of time (Lang and Lazovik, 1963). Stress levels remain low, and the horse should not be moved to the next level of exposure until it is comfortable with the one it is experiencing. If the animal does experience heightened levels of stress, it is suggested to retreat down the fear hierarchy and wait until stress is reduced once again (Christensen *et al.*, 2006). An example might be the introduction of a saddle and girth (Fig. 1.23), where over a period of time the horse is introduced to the weight and feel of the tack, rather than putting on the saddle and girth straight away and letting the horse habituate to the novel experience.

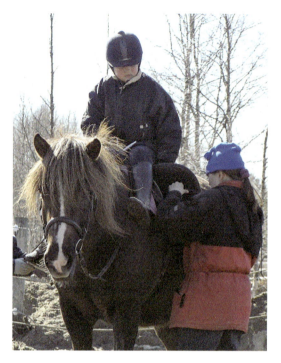

Fig. 1.23. Desensitization is used frequently. In this case the horse has been trained to accept the pressure of the girth.

Overshadowing

The process of overshadowing in learning theory has been explained in research and used with success in horses (McLean, 2008). The method involves the application of two different stimuli at the same time, which results in the stronger stimulus 'overshadowing' the weaker one, and the horse habituating to this weaker one, causing it to be extinguished (McLean and Christensen, 2017). This appears to be an extremely useful method of training for horses, particularly when the horse has learnt a leading action such as walking forward and backing up when asked by using pressure-release on the head-collar rope as negative reinforcement. This procedure of leading can then be used as the stronger stimulus in cases where the horse may be fearful over its environment, whether this may be the audience clapping at a show or the sound of clippers (Fig. 1.24).

Counter-conditioning

This method involves the training of an animal to perform a behaviour that is contradictory to the one that must be removed (McLean and Christensen, 2017). It is used with systematic desensitization to promote a desirable situation where stress is lessened, in a situation where the horse previously felt tension. For example, a horse

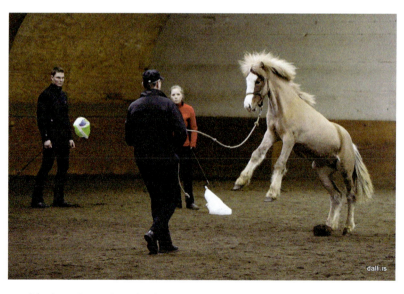

Fig. 1.24. Care must be taken when training fearful horses – this pony may well eventually habituate to the plastic bag, but how much stress has it had to suffer?

may well be fearful of motorbikes, perhaps due to a previous experience where it was frightened by the noise of one. Using counter-conditioning the arrival of an aversive motorbike could be paired with the handler asking the horse to perform a known behaviour such as target training. Ultimately the horse learns that the arrival of the motorbike is not worth reacting to and the fearful anticipation of the event is erased.

Generalization

Horses are rather unique in their domesticated companionship status with humans as, unlike dogs and cats, they are prey animals (Brubaker and Udell, 2016). They therefore have in their behavioural repertoire the ability to learn by generalization, not normally shared by predators in the animal kingdom. If adulthood is to be reached, a prey animal needs to learn very quickly what is a threat and what is not, thus the ability to generalize across similar objects such as types of predator to indicate that a quick departure is needed (Mitchell

et al., 2015). Therefore, when training a horse to walk into a trailer the handler may be surprised that the same horse will enter different trailers without having extra training for each design (Fig. 1.25). It is this ability that often allows surprising observations in horses when exposed to different trainers and riders – the horse appears to accept these differences without extra exposure and to respond well to many diverse humans although of dissimilar capability (Fureix *et al.*, 2009b).

The usefulness of having a horse that rarely responds to traffic is an example of this ability to generalize. Horses in their foundation training will be exposed to various vehicles when ridden, or otherwise taken out to experience traffic, and it can be observed that they will quickly generalize across many different types. Problems can arise when unexpected situations occur, such as a car backfiring or a very loud motorcycle passing at speed. These individual learnt experiences may then need to be modified with appetitive rewards and the young horse again exposed to other vehicles to advance its learning.

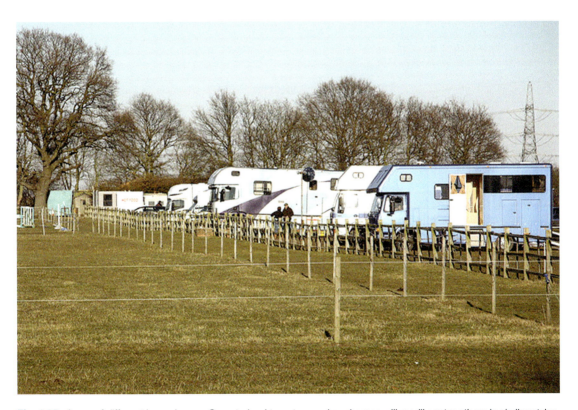

Fig. 1.25. A row of different horse boxes. Once trained to enter one box, horses will readily enter others in similar styles.

The Emergence of Equitation Science

Introduction

The beginnings of the study of learning theory in the horse first appeared in the mid-1980s, and increased rapidly in the 1990s. Many experiments concerning the application of learning theory in the training and management of horses occurred in this time period (Cooper, 1998; Mills, 1998), and the equine community began to talk about the beginnings of a new method of quantifying training techniques. This would act to improve the relationship and communication of horse and rider, effectively using learning theory as a training tool with the ultimate goal of improving equine welfare. Horses were no longer to be discussed in anthropomorphic terms (human emotions assigned to horses), or blame put on them for what was most likely the fault of the handler in misinterpreting the natural behaviour of the animal involved (Goodwin, 1999).

One of the first areas to be explored was that of stereotypies and their relationship to performance and welfare, where horses will perform seemingly pointless repeating behaviours for no obvious reason (McGreevy and Nicol, 1998). An example is crib-biting (where the horse will grab on to a protruding surface and sound as if it is swallowing air) (Fig. 1.26). These varied learnt behaviours were labelled 'vices', categorizing the problem as the horse's fault, when it is now known they generally arise from incorrect husbandry. The myth of horses copying these behaviours from one to another has also now been refuted (Nicol, 1999; Rorvang *et al.*, 2018), but multiple horses performing stereotypical behaviours on the same yard indicates welfare problems with their husbandry, not that they are displaying observational learning. Therefore, by modifying the way we keep our horses, many of these stereotypies can be prevented from happening, although it is to be noted that preventing those horses already displaying stereotypies by the many popular means such as using 'cribbing

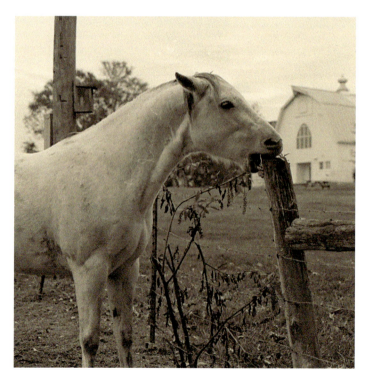

Fig. 1.26. A horse performing the stereotypy known as 'crib-biting' – it bites onto a surface and arches its neck to make a grunting sound.

collars' or electric shocks can actually cause the individual more stress (Briefer Freymond *et al.*, 2015).

The earliest mentions of equitation science in the literature came in the mid-2000s, where the idea was introduced in a scientific publication (McGreevy, 2007). The concept was described as a combination of the use of learning theory, ethology and physics aimed at understanding and measuring horse-training techniques. These measures were intended to target welfare aspects of training techniques, with the ultimate purpose of providing a scientific evidence-based comment to inform those working with horses how they could improve their practices. Since then, research in equitation science has explored many different areas of horse training, including the issue of tight nosebands (Docherty *et al.*, 2017), rein tension (Christensen *et al.*, 2011b) and saddle pressure (Greve and Dyson, 2013).

Investigation of physical indicators

Measures to investigate the welfare issues surrounding bridles and saddles have developed with great speed since the advent of equitation science, where stride length was first measured as imprints of hooves in a sand arena and evolved to gait analysis with laptops and the use of 'apps'. The progression of materials to measure pressure and tension have been avidly investigated by equitation scientists, keen to have methods to record objective data and process meaningful statistical analysis (Fig. 1.27). Perception of the rider's signals to the horse can now be measured, and sometimes compared with the familiar evaluation of stress by heart rate monitoring (Figs 1.28 and 1.29) and cortisol levels from

blood, urine or saliva. Contrasting or looking for correlation of measures in experiments allows scientists to investigate which methods to measure welfare might be best, and how they may perhaps interact. The observation of behaviour along with the physical study of heart rate, cortisol and pressures can provide an even more detailed picture of poor welfare in the horse.

Tallying behaviour

Objective tallying of behaviour in animals has long been used as a method to gauge stress, and ethograms have been designed to enable observers to log each behaviour seen as correctly as is possible. The equitation scientist, although not necessarily a trained ethologist, can readily use an ethogram to obtain behavioural information (Banks, 1982). Specific ethograms are currently being created and prototypes used for observation of the horse and rider partnership (Dyson *et al.*, 2018; Dyson, 2019). Many different behaviours can be recorded – such as ear movement, tail swishes, bucking – and also the frequency, latency and strength of the behaviour may be noted (Fig. 1.30). Video recordings can also be utilized to support ethogram tallying and to enable the accurate observation of behaviour. These methods have all elevated behavioural observation as a reliable method of welfare indication, and certainly with the ridden horse have explored the phenomenon of conflict behaviour.

Conflict behaviour

As previously discussed, the method of using negative reinforcement in training horses correctly relies

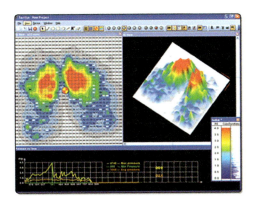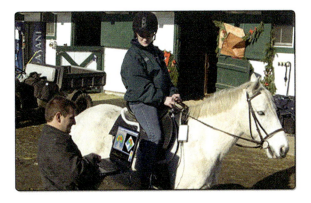

Fig. 1.27. Saddle pressure device, feeding back real-time information to a laptop computer (courtesy of Sensorprod.com).

upon the accurately timed release of pressure (Fenner *et al.*, 2017). If timings are used correctly, this reduces the occurrence of what is termed conflict behaviour and improves training (McLean, 2004). An example of where timing in riding is crucial would be in the schooling movement of a half-halt where the horse is asked to either slow down and speed up, or vice versa, in order to concentrate its

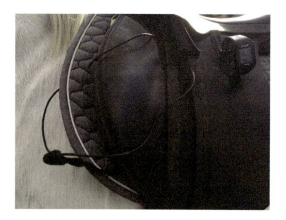

Fig. 1.28. A simple heart rate monitor can be used for lungeing or in-hand work with the Bluetooth® watch attached to the saddle.

attention back to the rider. Problems occur when the two signals are given simultaneously, confusing the horse as to whether it should slow down or speed up. This manifests in conflict behaviour, which can be seen commonly as a swift and rapid tail movement (Fig. 1.31), often named in journal papers as a 'tail swish' or 'tail lash' (Heleski *et al.*, 2009). The horse exhibits its confusion by tail swishing, and indeed in British dressage rules it is advised that judges mark down horses showing this behaviour (Fig. 1.32). Therefore, many investigations in the field of equitation science use behavioural observation, and a key factor amongst these is the tallying of conflict behaviour amongst the cohort in the experiment when observed for indicators of poor welfare.

The use of both physical and psychological factors features in the study of equitation science, and often a combination of the two are seen in research. The published literature covering many aspects of learning theory combined with the knowledge of ethology act as a tool through equitation science to endeavour to train horses correctly and appropriately to avoid problems developing in the first instance. Horses trained in this way make for a safer environment for both animal and human, where the knowledge of how horses react to different situations makes

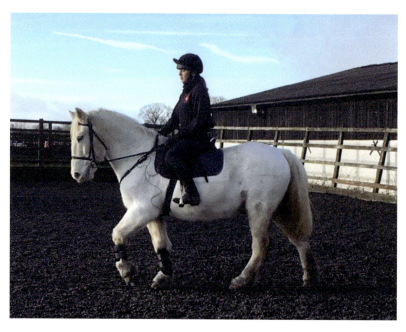

Fig. 1.29. A heart rate monitor used in ridden work, attached to the breastplate with the first pad under the saddle near the withers, and the second underneath the girth.

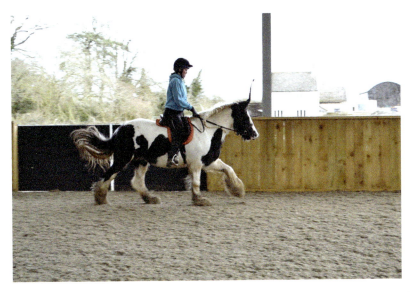

Fig. 1.30. Tallying behaviour – tail swishes, head movement and placement of ears can all be counted in frequency, duration or strength.

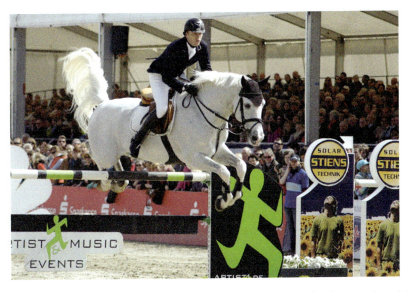

Fig. 1.31. The tail swish – seen as a rapid movement of the tail either upwards, downwards or laterally or a combination of all three.

for more aware and proficient handlers (Starling *et al.*, 2016). However, when training methods have failed, or inappropriate ridden and groundwork methods have taken place, equitation science can provide equine behaviourists with the tools to scrutinize problems, discover their origin if possible and ultimately to try to solve them.

The present – equitation science elucidating natural horsemanship

Equitation science has emerged into an equine world of traditionalism and the phenomenon of natural horsemanship. Traditional training techniques are supported with societies across the globe, where examinations and courses are available for riders and handlers to gain qualifications in all aspects of the equestrian field. Natural horsemanship, however, covers a vast array of different techniques intended to be a kinder way of dealing with horses (Goodwin *et al.*, 2009). Even though methods involved in natural horsemanship are sometimes very different, many rely on using

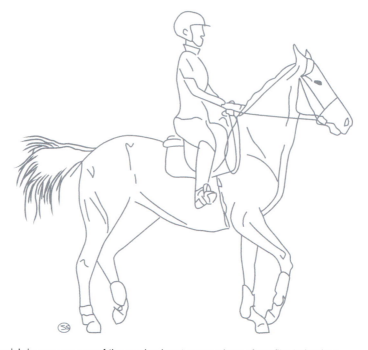

Fig. 1.32. The tail swish is seen as one of the predominant expressions of conflict behaviour.

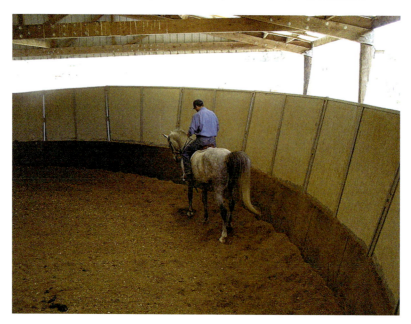

Fig. 1.33. A horse being ridden in a round-pen – this one has solid panels around the perimeter. (Montanabw.)

leadership/dominance models over the horse and attempt to use the submissive role to coerce horses into accepting the human's authority. This is problematic due to the concept of such leadership, as horses in a herd do not rely on a set hierarchy or dominant/submissive roles in their communication (McGreevy *et al.*, 2009).

Investigations into natural horsemanship techniques looking at pinpointing what learning processes are being used generally identify methods using negative reinforcement and punishment. Round-pen training (Fig. 1.33), where the horse is chased around a small circular area until it stops and turns in towards the handler, is seen as a submissive act, particularly if the horse shows licking and chewing behaviours. This can be interpreted incorrectly as signs of submission, whereas licking, chewing and yawning are actually signs of stress in horses (Warren-Smith and McGreevy, 2008; Górecka-Bruzda *et al.*, 2016). These signs of stress in the round-pen could be attributed to the incorrect use of negative reinforcement, where the handler does not allow the horse a release of pressure when it is running around the pen. This pressure is sometimes applied by a rope, or a lunge whip, and if this pressure is not removed/released to reward the horse then it ceases to be negative reinforcement and becomes punishment (Baragli *et al.*, 2015; Kydd *et al.*, 2017). When the handler using round-pen techniques does move away from the horse, and reduces the pressure, this is then negatively reinforced, and the horse learns to slow down/stop and interact (McGreevy *et al.*, 2009). It is possible to misinterpret this as a leadership contest, but by applying learning theory it can be seen clearly that this is training and understanding in progress.

Other methods of natural horsemanship also rely on the leadership/dominance model, such as those that have set games or training periods where the handler uses different approaches to gain the 'trust' of the horse or dominance over it. Many of these use ropes and long whips to 'ask' the horse to move in certain directions, and again these are often misconstrued and sometimes even labelled as positive reinforcement. Each time pressure is used it is negatively reinforcing the movement, and if the pressure is not removed, it becomes punishment; therefore the misunderstanding of the use of negative reinforcement is commonly seen in these techniques. Certainly, many of these game techniques are very anthropomorphic in their titles alone, suggesting that horses understand the basic concepts of trust, respect and friendship. Currently no evidence exists for the understanding of these terms by horses, and the language of anthropomorphism is common where humans condemn certain sports that use horses (Legg *et al.*, 2019). Indeed, using such words can lay the blame on the horse, for being 'naughty' or 'mistrustful', when it is using what is termed by humans as undesirable behaviour due to stress or pain. Therefore, it is extremely easy to misinterpret a horse's behaviour if handlers do equate horses with human emotions, and certainly a dubious path to follow if investigating these behaviours.

Nevertheless, the tenets of natural horsemanship where knowledge of behaviour leads to better treatment are certainly worthy of inclusion in training, for example where horses are being treated as sentient rather than as objects to further human careers. If handlers and trainers aim to better themselves with education into horse behaviour, and watch their charges closely, this alone gives credence to some of the methods used. However, it is still extremely important that the handler understands exactly how the horse is learning, to avoid the behavioural problems that can arise in horses treated with what is thought to be kindness, when it is actually punishment.

Natural horsemanship is not, however, isolated in its misunderstanding of equine behaviour. Documents published by various equine societies regularly use anthropomorphic language and terms such as submission and obedience. When traditional practices have been in place for so long, it is tempting to leave them alone as they have always worked in the past, so why not continue? But the number of unwanted horses seen at slaughterhouses and charities may indicate problem behaviour that cannot be underestimated. Wastage of racehorses through behavioural problems is a known factor (Thompson *et al.*, 2014); misbehaviour is perceived as dangerous in 52% of cases in riding ponies (Buckley *et al.*, 2013); and behavioural responses such as separation anxiety in horses causes more injury occurrence (Owen *et al.*, 2012). These issues may indicate that traditional ways of training must be improved, or at the least understood and adapted to current scientific thinking.

A note on basic groundwork

Many equine training programmes, including natural horsemanship, traditional methods and those techniques using learning theory, base their foundations on some type of groundwork. This may include lungeing, long-reining, free-schooling, or work in-hand with either bridle or headcollar. Each one commonly exists to prepare the young horse for ridden work, with signals and manoeuvres meant to emulate those used once the horse is mounted. However, when examining these through the lens of equitation science a rather different picture of what is happening can emerge.

The use of lungeing has been compared with round-pen training (Fenner *et al.*, 2019), which relies on chasing the horse to supposedly dominate it and accept the handler as its leader. Even though it has been discussed earlier that this is not actually happening, the same negative connotations with round-pen might be seen in lungeing if pressure is not released from the horse at the correct times. Until further research is done, there is concern that lungeing may possibly be reinforcing the flight response in the young horse if not used correctly. A horse that has been continually chased, either on the lunge or in the round-pen, may inadvertently use this hard-wired behaviour when it faces stressful situations in ridden work, leading to running away, commonly termed bolting. Advice is often given to novice riders that lungeing a horse before riding will act to make it 'calmer' or more settled; however, if the flight response is reinforced in this way it may contribute to more ridden problems, not fewer.

Long-reining by contrast attempts to emulate the rider's signals once mounted on the horse, therefore enabling the training of these signals to take place before the additional stress and weight of the rider. A bridle or lungeing cavesson is used, sometimes a plain headcollar, with two long lunge lines or reins attached one to each side of the bridle or other device. The handler trains the horse by negative reinforcement, asking it to walk on by agitating the lines on both its sides, comparative to where the legs will be positioned, and stopping this motion once the horse moves forward. Additionally, the horse is trained to stop with pressure on the lines, which should be released as soon as the horse slows to shape the response, and when it halts. For lateral movement, the lines are used individually as leg pressure would be: for movement to the left, the right line is agitated, pressure is put on the left line and vice versa. It is obviously imperative for learning that the pressure in all instances is released once the horse responds. The expert 'long-reiner' can

become very efficient in the use of the lines, and young horses learn readily using this method.

Free-schooling is used in different ways, but generally in an enclosed school or arena. Futurity or grading events, where sports horses are awarded certain points for various physical conformations, sometimes use free-schooling along marked channels in an arena to better observe the dynamic movement of the horse in question. Jumps can also be positioned in the channels, leaving the horse no choice but to go over them. Before the event the horses are usually trained in the same manner; however, once lunge whips or lines are used to persuade the horse to trot or canter and jump, the handler risks using punishment if pressure from these tools is not removed to negatively reinforce the behaviour. In these forms of groundwork, no published research to date has been carried out to determine how unwanted behaviours might develop with these systems, but learning theory can certainly be understood in this context to warrant careful use of these methods of training.

Conversely, groundwork involving a single handler and horse using a bridle or headcollar has been documented when studying reinforcement in experiments (Murphy and Arkins, 2007). Target training as a precursor to loading problematic horses used negative reinforcement (Ferguson and Rosales-Ruiz, 2001), positive reinforcement with frightening situations (Heleski *et al.*, 2008) and combinations of the two types of reinforcement (Valenchon *et al.*, 2017). Horses do respond well to reinforcement training, and both types as discussed appear to work well. When training a horse to lead, both methods are used through the various training techniques, but the timing of pressure-release must be accurate when using negative reinforcement, as stated before.

Training a horse to lead through this type of reinforcement would start with the horse learning to move towards the handler only when pressure is applied to the lead rope, and to stop in the same way. Timing is crucial to provide the reward, and shaping can be used when the horse trials the correct behaviour. Horses that have been trained in traditional methods without the pressure-release or with positive reinforcement tend to learn to follow the handler. However, in circumstances where the handler wants the horse to stand still for veterinary treatment or hoof work it is beneficial to have a horse that does not do this, but stands still waiting for pressure to signal it to move (Fig. 1.34). This is achieved by training the movement forwards and

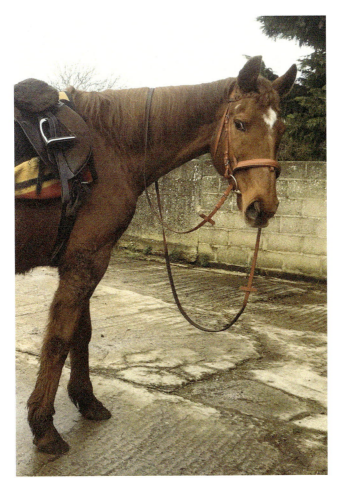

Fig. 1.34. Horse 'parked' – it will not move until pressure is applied to the reins.

backwards with pressure-release on the lead rope, and then by moving away from the horse and correcting any following behaviour by asking the horse to return to its starting position. Horses readily learn this technique, and if trained in this way they tend to generalize the training and improve in their ridden work.

Groundwork using both positive and negative reinforcement correctly acts as a suitable precursor to ridden work, in young horses and when retraining older horses that have problems with bolting, napping or other undesirable behaviours. Issues are raised when they are not used correctly and in the right circumstances. Certain methods can involve the use of a whip, sometimes as a substitute or additional signal to the pressure on the lead rope, or in others a long rope flicked at the head/neck of the horse to induce it

to move backwards. Again, care must be taken that the whip is used only as a signalling device, and removed once the horse moves in the direction it is being asked. With the long rope the problem is apparent in the continued use of the flicking motion when the horse is already reversing, thus not giving a reward and becoming punishment. Horses can react very badly to these methods, and psychological problems can develop (Hall *et al.*, 2008).

A note on stereotypies

Development of stereotypies is still not fully agreed upon, even after a large amount of research has been carried out (Briefer Freymond *et al.*, 2019). There are suggestions that can be made on evidence, however, and this subject is recommended for studying by anyone dealing with horses, as stereotypies are not necessarily uncommon and can affect welfare significantly.

In horses, stereotypies can be separated into two groups: those involved with movement, named locomotory; and those that are based around oral issues. Examples seen by horsepersons are the oral stereotypies of crib-biting and wind-sucking, and the locomotory stereotypies of box-walking and weaving. They are separated into these two groups due to their morphology, but also because their development tends to be from an oral or locomotory origin.

Since research has suggested that horses who are prevented from acting out stereotypies are more stressed (Briefer Freymond et al., 2015), it has been generally accepted that horses should be allowed to perform their stereotypies. This is also reflected in the discovery that horses probably do not have the capacity to learn by observation (Rorvang et al., 2018), explaining their inability to copy their counterparts. If horses living on the same yard display stereotypies, or others are brought in and develop them, it is due to poor husbandry and yard environment and not copying behaviour. As this has entered general knowledge, horses with stereotypies now tend not to be hidden away in separate stables and paddocks, which obviously works to their advantage by allowing the companionship that can help to alleviate their stress.

Oral stereotypies

These are thought to derive from appetitive restriction, for instance horses fed their ration of hay in the evening and it running out before midnight. This may leave the animal without any form of food, generally fibre, for quite a few hours, something not experienced in natural equine maintenance behaviour. Due to horses therefore needing to chew, many oral stereotypies can be traced back to the lack of fibre in their diet (Bachmann et al., 2003), where the motivation builds into frustration and the horse will use any oral stimulation to satisfy its needs. Other factors influence this, such as the process of weaning (Waters et al., 2002), turnout time (Christie et al., 2006) and lack of tactile contact with other horses (Bachmann et al., 2003). For example, horses bedded on straw rather than shavings tend to develop fewer oral stereotypies (Christie et al., 2006), probably due to the availability of the bedding to have a chew on when their hay or haylage runs out.

Locomotory stereotypies

This class of stereotypy originates in the restriction of movement, which is of course an essential behaviour for the horse as a prey animal. Weaving and box-walking are forms of alleviation of the inability to roam whilst confined in a stable, and perfectly understandable when it has been reported that feral horses travel approximately 16 km a day (Hampson et al., 2010). Horses confined to stables have completely different time budgets to feral horses, spending a large amount of their time standing still in comparison with their wide-ranging counterparts. Interestingly, types of locomotory stereotypies can be correlated with discipline (McGreevy et al., 1995); for example, dressage horses tend to display more overall than eventers or endurance horses, but the latter display more box-walking. Treating them might seem easier than oral types; however, those horses conditioned deeply to perform their stereotypies have been known to weave in fields by entrance gates.

Stereotypies – can we treat them?

Solving issues around stereotypies historically involved stopping the horse from carrying out the behaviour. Examples exist such as foul-tasting gum spread on stable doors to stop chewing and electronic devices to shock the horse if they try to bite the surface or kick the door. The leather cribbing collar, where a fixed spike was used to dig into the jawline to deter the physical action of crib-biting, was quite popular to use on horses at one time. Weaving bars are still used extensively to try to prevent the exaggerated movement characteristics of this stereotypy, but they generally fail to achieve their objective, with the horse moving inside the stable and carrying on weaving. Welfare advancements and improved education have now tended to stop these practices, although they can still be seen on some yards in the UK.

Currently, prevention is an improvement of attempting to solve the stereotypy, and measures taken particularly with weaning and husbandry can help to alleviate the number of horses developing them. There are methods that can be used to lessen the behaviours, including increasing fibre availability, turnout to expand exercise and natural behaviours and changes of routine in husbandry in general. Unfortunately practices of weaning are very traditional, though some yards have trialled new methods such as natural weaning (Morel et al.,

2007), where the foals are kept with the natal band until they instinctively stop feeding, and keeping the foals with other mares to offer a nursery-type system. If these practices prove to increase profitability or performance, there is a possibility of them being brought into standard preparation.

A quick introduction to horse psychology

Stress and fear – measurement and confusion

Stress is the body's answer to the challenge of returning its systems back to the norm after an experience such as psychological pressure, injury or exercise (Wagner, 2010). Acute stress occurs in a single episode, and does not cause long-term harm; however, when a series of acute stresses occurs without relief this can develop into a chronic condition. Psychological stress can be a cause of behavioural problems brought on by anxiety in certain situations, particularly where fear plays a part.

Fear itself is a physiological, behavioural and emotional reaction to situational stimuli that the horse encounters and manifests as prey preparation for flight or fight. These can include physical reactions, such as raised heart rate and pacing, and behavioural consequences, such as a heightened level of perception. Behaviours could include displacement/redirected behaviours, destructive behaviours and excessive vocalization. The level displayed may be affected by the individual's previous experience, characteristics of the type of stimulus and whether the animal is cornered or restrained. This leads to a state of frustration, where motivation is hindered, and problems begin to develop.

It is important as part of equine research to measure stress correctly. This is fraught with difficulty, as the methods used do not always align with each other, and certainly in some cases are far more problematic to measure accurately than is realized. The standard methods of measuring stress include cortisol (blood, saliva, or in bodily waste), heart rate/heart rate variation (HR/HRV), and behavioural observation (most commonly conflict behaviour). Each method has its own set of problems, and can be exacerbated by the use of cheap measuring tools, collection protocol and variations in ethograms. As stated, the problem of corroboration appears very pertinent, as horses that are experiencing damaging psychological states of mind, such as learned helplessness, may not even display normal signs of stress due to the condition itself (Konig von Borstel et al., 2017).

Frustration and motivation

Anticipatory behaviours are those that develop from the motivational need to perform maintenance behaviours – those of eating, drinking, running, staying in a herd, for example – and the frustration caused when the horse is prevented from doing so (Peters et al., 2012). Examples of these might be striking out, pawing, biting and other problems experienced in a restrictive environment. This concept of frustration in horses is possibly the most common underlying factor in the development of behavioural problems, where the horse is motivated to carry out an action, but the handler/rider aims to prevent it doing so. This can be displayed as physical force (from the handler/rider), by decision (the horse is undecided or confused about what action to take) or where the animal is thwarted in what it is trying to do (food is visible but is unobtainable) (Manning and Dawkins, 2012). As the horse continues to try to perform the behaviour that would normally lead it to the goal of its motivation, it

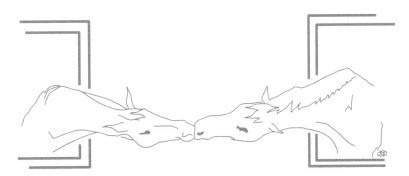

Fig. 1.35. Even stabled horses need contact with others – it is a pronounced motivating force.

becomes trapped in an appetitive phase, which is very hard to break (Fig. 1.35).

Redirected behaviours are slightly different. An example might be a horse that is stabled, with other horses being led past it: the horse wants to follow but is prevented from doing so and performs the behaviour in the only direction it can, in this case the start of box-walking. Others may react in different ways, such as beginning to sway in the door, and begin to develop weaving. Behaviours such as these are named redirected behaviours, because the motivation is directed to something else, so the example above where movement towards another horse is prevented progresses into box-walking (Goodwin *et al.*, 2002). Displacement behaviour occurs through the same frustrating situations but involves seemingly meaningless or unrelated behaviour such as biting a surface or indeed itself. Even the inexperienced behaviourist can now see where this might happen, and how in fact anyone involved with the daily care of horses is inadvertently 'training' them continuously to respond to different stimuli, ultimately leading to behavioural problems.

Two examples of chronic stress disorders

Conditioned suppression is a response to the horse learning to supress its motivation in an attempt to stop whatever is happening to it, for example jabbing in the mouth when the rider becomes unbalanced. This involves a conditioned emotional response with its root in fear, so the horse learns that the jab in the mouth, which causes fear, cannot be escaped. The horse ceases to respond to the jabs and can seem to be a perfect 'schoolmaster', whereas it has become dull and unresponsive through habituation. In horses the incorrect use of negative reinforcement (frequent, unavoidable and aversive) can lead to the same withdrawn dull state where the horse will never attempt more than it needs to – and does not show any initiative, producing the well-known schoolmaster example.

Learned helplessness is also a psychological condition occurring through incorrect negative reinforcement, though it is different in its expression. If an animal learns that it has no control over an aversive stimulus, it may give up attempting to escape from that stimulus (Hall *et al.*, 2008). In dogs this was demonstrated using an electric shock chamber, where the animal could not escape from the shock whatever behaviour it trialled and eventually

became completely unresponsive (Seligman and Maier, 1967). The common phrases heard in the equine world of a horse having a 'hard mouth' or one that is 'dead to the leg' can be explained with learned helplessness. In the first case the rider is not using negative reinforcement correctly and may be continuing to pull on the reins once the horse has slowed, or in the second case where the rider is kicking regardless of whether the horse is speeding up or not. Each situation involves the horse learning that it has no control over the pulling and/or kicking, and it cannot escape the pain, so it becomes unresponsive. An example might be the riding school pony, who is labelled as 'lazy' and is reluctant to move forward even when kicked continuously or a whip is brought into action. The pony may simply have given up and knows through experience that it cannot escape from the rider's actions, and therefore is not motivated to move or indeed even stop.

A simple test thought to indicate to owners and handlers if a horse might be suffering from learned helplessness is commonly called the 'carrot and bucket test', where a horse in its stable is shown a carrot being placed under an upturned unfamiliar bucket. The latency of approach to and seeking of the carrot is then measured, and it is noted if the carrot is uncovered (Fig. 1.36). There have been no published data to corroborate the usefulness of this task, but it has been used anecdotally to evaluate polo ponies, as their husbandry differs to that for other sports horses regarding turnout and group living (Duncan, 2019). It may be that future research might investigate further the phenomenon of learned helplessness and the usefulness of such tests in discovering if welfare issues exist in certain populations of horses.

The role of the equine behaviourist

Equine behaviour problems in the UK appear to exist in very high numbers, with one study reporting 91% of owners recording ridden problems in their horses (Hockenhull and Creighton, 2013). The most dangerous ridden problems of rearing and bolting were seen in 7% and 3% of horses, respectively; this seems like a low number at first but nonetheless is still very much a cause for concern. Also, the ability of horsepersons to recognize behavioural distress in horses is very low (Fig. 1.37), and this is extremely worrying for the welfare of horses in the UK (Bell *et al.*, 2019).

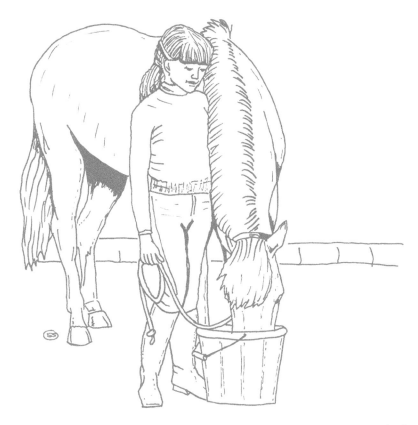

Fig. 1.36. Horses suffering from learned helplessness will sometimes not even try to turn over a bucket, even if they have seen the carrot placed there and can smell it.

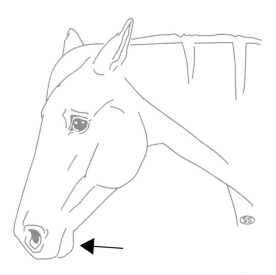

Fig. 1.37. It is not necessarily easy to spot the subtle signs of a distressed horse, such as this small upwards and inwards placing of the chin, combined with a wrinkled eye and ears held slightly caudal to the body.

At present no qualifications are required to practise as any form of behaviourist and there exists no regulatory body in the UK that they must belong to. This means that the profession includes many people who have no qualifications or even a basic understanding of learning theory and the science behind behaviour. Therefore, it is entirely the decision of the owner who to engage for their horse's problem but it is highly advised that they consult their veterinary surgeon to find a behaviourist, as they will know of recommended and qualified people. In addition to this, owners should always consult their vet, as many cases of problem behaviour do involve the horse developing the response as a result of pain or discomfort (Jonckheer-Sheehy *et al.*, 2012). The horse will ideally have a full examination before a behaviourist attends and will also benefit from having its tack checked by professionals. A competent behaviourist will always ask if the vet has been called out and will often suggest that this is done before they attend.

A full, detailed history should be taken, so that a thorough understanding of the environment the horse is living in can be considered if needed. Information on feeding, stabling/turnout, previous medical conditions and herd companions may all add substance to the overall diagnosis of the problem behaviour. Previous history, owners and any other disciplines undertaken can also give clues to working out the aetiology of the problem. The behaviourist will then watch the owner or handler closely and determine how they handle the animal, the condition of the communication between the two and any other observations that could prove useful. Placing the horse in the position of acting out the problem behaviour is preferred for examination, but in some cases it is not necessary, due to the preliminary observation or because the behaviour is too dangerous to repeat.

One visit is generally enough to devise an action plan or a retraining programme, but it is worth bearing in mind that other visits may be appropriate to check on improvement and possibly advise further or change the method or techniques if suited to the horse's progression. A professional behaviourist likes to see the conclusion of their work and may arrange to visit the horse at no cost while on another round to see the results. Owners also need to make sure they inform their behaviourist of any changes, either behavioural or to the environment the horse is in, in case this might affect their retraining programme. Even small changes might be very important, so it is worth noting these down and communicating them to the behaviourist.

The behavioural problems, key points and take-home messages in the following chapters come from authentic scenarios, where equitation science with its basis in learning theory is used to solve real-life equine challenges. The case studies are reported from various visits in the past, but do not include names, correct breeds of horses or identifying factors. It must be stated the book is intended as a guide to those wishing to discover more about equine behaviour problems and solutions to solve them using science but is not a substitute for a professional behaviourist attending to a horse with challenges.

References

Ahrendt, L.P., Labouriaub, R., Malmkvist, J., Nicole, C.J. and Christensen, J.W. (2015) Development of a standard test to assess negative reinforcement learning in horses. *Applied Animal Behaviour Science* 169, 38–42.

Bachmann, I., Audige, L. and Stauffacher, M. (2003) Risk factors associated with behavioural disorders of crib-biting, weaving and box-walking in Swiss horses. *Equine Veterinary Journal* 35(2), 158–163.

Banks, E.M. (1982) Behavioural research to answer questions about animal welfare. *Journal of Animal Science* 54(2), 434–446.

Baragli, P., Padalino, B. and Telatin, A. (2015) The role of associative and non-associative learning in the training of horses and implications for the welfare (a review). *Annali dell'Instituto superior di sanita* 51(1), 40–51.

Bell, C., Rogers, S., Taylor, J. and Busby, D. (2019) Improving the recognition of Equine Affective States. *Animals (Basel)* 9(12), e1124.

Bradshaw, G. (2009) Looking out: neuroethological compromise effects of elephants in captivity. In: Forthman, D.L., Kane, L.F., Hancocks, D. and Waldau, P.F. (eds) *An Elephant in the Room*. Tufts Center for Animals and Public Policy, North Grafton, Massachusetts.

Briefer Freymond, S., Bardou, D., Briefer, E.F., Bruckmaier, R., Fouche, N. *et al.* (2015) The physiological consequences of crib-biting in horses in response to an ACHT challenge test. *Physiological Behaviour* 151, 121–128.

Briefer Freymond, S., Ruet, A., Grivaz, M., Fuentes, C., Zuberbuehler, K. *et al.* (2019) Stereotypic horses (*Equus caballus*) are not cognitively impaired. *Animal Cognition* 22(1), 17–33.

Brollo, A. (2006) First steps of clicker training: targeting. Available at: https://commons.wikimedia.org/wiki/File:Horse_clicker_training_italy_2.jpg (Accessed 2 March 2020).

Brubaker, L. and Udell, M.A. (2016) Cognition and learning in horses (*Equus caballus*): what we know and why we should ask more. *Behavioural Processes* 126, 121–131.

Buckley, P., Morton, J.M., Buckley, D.J. and Coleman, G.T. (2013) Misbehaviour in Pony Club horses: incidence and risk factors. *Equine Veterinary Journal* 45(1), 9–14.

Cooper, J.J. (1998) Comparative learning theory and its application in the training of horses. *Equine Veterinary Journal (Supplement)* 27, 39–43.

Christensen, J.W. (2013) Object habituation in horses: the effect of voluntary versus negatively reinforced approach to frightening stimuli. *Equine Veterinary Journal* 45(3), 298–301.

Christensen, J.W., Rundgren, M. and Olsson, K. (2006) Training methods for horses: habituation to a frightening stimulus. *Equine Veterinary Journal* 38(5), 439–443.

Christensen, J.W., Sondergaard, E., Thodberga, K. and Halekoh, U. (2011a) Effects of repeated regrouping on horse behaviour and injuries. *Applied Animal Behaviour Science* 133(3-4), 199–206.

Christensen, J.W., Zharkikh, T.L., Antoine, A. and Malmkvist, J. (2011b) Rein tension acceptance in young horses in a voluntary test situation. *Equine Veterinary Journal* 43(2), 223–228.

Christie, J.L., Hewson, C.J., Riley, C.B., McNiven, M.A., Dohoo, I.R. and Bate, L.A. (2006) Management factors affecting stereotypies and body condition score in non-racing horses in Prince Edward Island. *Canadian Veterinary Journal* 47(2), 136–143.

Claussen, G. and Hessel, E.F. (2017) Particulate matter in equestrian stables and riding areas. *Journal of Equine Veterinary Science* 55, 67–70.

Cowdery, G.E., Iwata, B.A. and Pace, G.M. (1990) Effects and side effects of DRO as treatment for self-injurious behavior. *Journal of Applied Behaviour Analysis* 23(4), 497–506.

Craig, D.P.A., Varnon, C.A., Pollock, K.L. and Abramson, C.I. (2015) An assessment of horse (*Equus ferrus caballus*) responding on fixed interval schedules of reinforcement: an individual analysis. *Behavioural Processes* 120, 1–13.

Docherty, O., Casey, V., McGreevy, P. and Arkins, S. (2017) Noseband use in equestrian sports – an international study. *PLoS ONE* 12(1).

Duncan, S. (2019) A study into the prevalence of 'learned helplessness' within a polo pony population. BSc (Hons), Oxford Brookes University, Oxford.

Dyson, S. (2019) Application of a ridden horse ethogram to horses competing at a 4-star three day event: comparison with cross-country performance. *Equine Veterinary Journal* 51, 553.

Dyson, S., Berger, J., Ellis, A. and Mullard, J. (2018) Development of an ethogram for a pain scoring system in ridden horses and its application to determine the presence of musculoskeletal pain. *Journal of Veterinary Behaviour: Clinical Applications and Research* 23, 47–57.

Ellis, D., Fell, M., Luck, K., Gill, L., Owen, H. *et al*. (2015) Effect of forage presentation on feed intake behaviour in stabled horses. *Applied Animal Behaviour Science* 165, 88–94.

Fenner, K., Webb, H., Starling, M.J., Freire, R., Buckley, P. and Greevy, P.D. (2017) Effects of pre-conditioning on behavior and physiology of horses during a standardised learning task. *PLoS ONE* 12(3).

Fenner, K., McLean, A.N. and McGreevy, P.D. (2019) Cutting to the chase: how round pen, lungeing and high-speed liberty work may compromise horse welfare. *Journal of Veterinary Behaviour* 29, 88–94.

Ferguson, D.L. and Rosales-Ruiz, J. (2001) Loading the problem loader: the effects of target training and shaping on trailer-loading behaviour of horses. *Journal of Applied Behaviour* 34(4), 409–423.

Ferster, C.B. and Skinner, B.F. (1957) *Schedules of Reinforcement*. Appleton-Century-Crofts, New York.

Fox, A.E., Bailey, S.R., Hall, E.G. and St Peter, C.C. (2012) Reduction of biting and chewing of horses using differential reinforcement of other behaviours. *Behavioural Processes* 91(1), 125–128.

Froehlich, D.J. (2002) Quo vadis eophippus? The systematics and taxonomy of the early Eocene equids (Perissodactyla). *Zoological Journal of the Linnean Society* 134(2), 141–256.

Fureix, C., Pages, M., Bon, R., Lassalle, J.M., Kuntz, P. and Gonzalez, G. (2009a) A preliminary study of the effects of handling type on horses' emotional reactivity and the human–horse relationship. *Behavioural Processes* 82(2), 202–210.

Fureix, C.I., Jego, P., Sankey, C. and Hausberger, M. (2009b) How horses (*Equus caballus*) see the world: humans as significant 'objects'. *Animal Cognition* 12(4), 643–654.

Glunk, E.C., Hathaway, M.R., Weber, W.J., Sheaffer, C.C. and Martinson, K.L. (2014) The effect of hay net design on rate of forage consumption when feeding adult horses. *Science* 34(8), 986–991.

Goodwin, D. (1999) The importance of ethology in understanding the behaviour of the horse. *Equine Veterinary Journal Supplement* (28), 15–19.

Goodwin, D., Davidson, H.P.B. and Harris, P. (2002) Foraging enrichment for stabled horses: effects on behaviour and selection. *Equine Veterinary Journal* 34(7), 686–691.

Goodwin, D., McGreevy, P., Waran, N. and McLean, A. (2009) How equitation science can elucidate and refine horsemanship techniques. *Veterinary Journal* 181(1), 5–11.

Górecka-Bruzda, A., Fureix, C., Ouvrard, A., Bourjade, M. and Hausberger, M. (2016) Investigating determinants of yawning in the Domestic (*Equus Caballus*) and Przewalski (*Equus Ferus Przewalskii*) Horses. *Naturwissenschaften* 103(9–10), 72.

Grandin, T. and Deesing, M.J. (2014) *Behavioral Genetics and Animal Science*, 2nd edn. Academic Press, London.

Greve, L. and Dyson, S. (2013) The horse-saddle-rider interaction. *Veterinary Journal* 195(3), 275–281.

Guay, K., Fuentes, M., Trice, R., Elmore, S., Attala, M. *et al*. (2019) Effects of level of bedding on lying behavior in stalled horses. *Journal of Equine Veterinary Science* 76, 122–123.

Hall, C., Goodwin, D., Heleski, C., Randle, H. and Waran, N. (2008) Is there evidence of learned helplessness in horses? *Journal of Applied Animal Welfare Science* 11(3), 249–266.

Hampson, B.A., de Laat, M.A., Mills, P.C. and Pollitt, C.C. (2010). Distances travelled by feral horses in 'outback' Australia. *Equine Veterinary Journal (Supplement)* 38, 582–586.

Hartman, N. and Greening, L.M. (2019). A preliminary study investigating the influence of auditory stimulation on the occurrence of nocturnal equine sleep-related behavior in stabled horses. *Journal of Equine Veterinary Science* 82, e102782.

Hartmann, E., Christensen, J.W. and McGreevy, P.D. (2017) Dominance and leadership: useful concepts in human–horse interactions? *Journal of Equine Veterinary Science* 52, 1–9.

Heath, S. and Wilson, C. (2014) Canine and feline enrichment in the home and kennel: a guide for practitioners. *Veterinary Clinics of North America: Small Practice* 44(3), 427–449.

Heleski, C., Bauson, L. and Bello, N. (2008) Evaluating the addition of positive reinforcement for learning a frightening task: a pilot study with horses. *Journal of Applied Animal Welfare Science* 11(3), 213–222.

Heleski, C., McGreevy P.D. and Clayton, H.M. (2009) Effects on behaviour and rein tension on horses ridden with or without martingales and rein inserts. *Veterinary Journal* 181(1), 56–62.

Henderson J.V. and Waran, N.K. (2001) Reducing equine stereotypies using an Equiball™. *Animal Welfare* 10, 73–80.

Hendriksen, P., Elmgreen, K. and Ladewig, J. (2010) Trailer loading of horses: is there a difference in positive and negative reinforcement concerning effectiveness and stress-related symptoms? *Journal of Veterinary Behavior* 5(4), 215–216.

Henry, S., Fureix, C., Rowberry, R., Bateson, M. and Hausberger, M. (2017). Do horses with poor welfare show 'pessimistic' cognitive biases? *Naturwissenschaften* 104(1–2), 8.

Hockenhull, J. and Creighton, E. (2013) The use of equipment and training practices and the prevalence of owner-reported ridden behaviour problems in UK leisure horses. *Equine Veterinary Journal* 45(1), 15–19.

Hockenhull, J. and Creighton, E. (2014) Management practices associated with owner-reported stable-related and handling behaviour problems in UK leisure horses. *Applied Animal Behaviour Science* 155, 49–55.

Innes, L. and McBride, S. (2008) Negative versus positive reinforcement: an evaluation of training strategies for rehabilitated horses. *Applied Animal Behaviour Science* 112(3-4), 357–368.

Jonckheer-Sheehy, V.S.M., Delesalle, C.J., van den Belt, A.J.M. and den Boom, R. (2012) Bad behaviour or a physical problem? Rearing in a Dutch Warmblood mare. *Journal of Veterinary Behavior* 7(6), 380–385.

Keeling, L.J., Boeb, K.E., Christensen, J.W., Hyyppad, S., Janssone, H. *et al.* (2016) Injury incidence, reactivity and ease of handling of horses kept in groups: a matched case control study in four Nordic countries. *Applied Animal Behaviour Science* 185, 59–65.

Konig von Borstel, U., Visser, E.K. and Hall, C. (2017) Indicators of stress in equitation. *Applied Animal Behaviour Science* 190, 43–56.

Kwiatkowska-Stenzel, A., Sowinska, J. and Witkowska, D. (2016) The effect of different bedding materials used in stable on horses' behaviour. *Journal of Equine Veterinary Science* 42, 57–66.

Kydd, E., Padalino, B., Henshall, C. and McGreevy, P. (2017) An analysis of equine round pen training videos

posted online: differences between amateur and professional trainers. *PLoS ONE* 12(9).

Lang, P.J. and Lazovik, A.D. (1963) Experimental desensitization of phobia. *Journal of Abnormal and Social Psychology* 66(6), 519.

Lau, A.N., Peng, L., Goto, H, Chemnick, L., Ryder, O.A. and Makova, K.D. (2009) Horse domestication and conservation genetics of Przewalski's Horse inferred from sex chromosomal and autosomal sequence. *Molecular Biology and Evolution* 26(1), 199–208.

LeDoux, J.E. (1994) Emotion, memory and the brain. *Scientific American* 270(6), 50–57.

Legg, K.A., Breheny, M., Gee, E.K. and Rogers, C.W. (2019) Responding to risk: regulation or prohibition? New Zealand Media reporting of Thoroughbred jumps racing 2016–2018. *Animals (Basel)* 9(5), 276.

Le Simple, C., Reverchon-Billota, L., Galloux, P., Stompa, M., Boichot, L. *et al.* (2020) Free movement: a key welfare improvement in sport horses? *Applied Animal Behavioural Science* [in press].

Losonci, Z. and Paddison, B.J. (2016) Do stabled horses show more undesirable behaviors during handling than field-kept ones? *Journal of Veterinary Behaviour* 15, 93.

Manning, M.S. and Dawkins, A. (2012) *An Introduction to Animal Behaviour*, 6th edn. Cambridge University Press, Cambridge.

McAfee, L.M., Mills, D. and Cooper, J.J. (2002) The use of mirrors for the control of stereotypic weaving behaviour in the stabled horse. *Applied Animal Behaviour Science* 78(2–4), 159–173.

Mills, D.S. (1998) Applying learning theory to the management of the horse: the difference between getting it right and getting it wrong. *Equine Veterinary Journal (Supplement)* 27, 44–48.

Mitchell, M.D., Chivers, D.P., McCormick, M.I. and Ferrari, M.C.O. (2015) Learning to distinguish between predators and non-predators: understanding the critical role of diet cues and predator odours in generalisation. *Scientific Reports* 5, 13918.

McFadden, B.J. (2005) Fossil horses – evidence for evolution. *Science* 307(5716), 1728–1730.

McGreevy, P.D. (2007) The advent of equitation science. *Veterinary Journal* 174(3), 492–500.

McGreevy, P.D. and Nicol, C.J. (1998) Prevention of cribbiting: a review. *Equine Veterinary Journal (Supplement)* 27, 35–38.

McGreevy, P.D., French, N.P. and Nicol, C.J. (1995) The prevalence of abnormal behaviours in dressage, eventing and endurance horses in relation to stabling. *Veterinary Record* 137(2), 36–37.

McGreevy, P.D., Oddie, C., Burton, F.L. and McLean, A.N. (2009) The horse–human dyad: can we align horse training and handling activities with the equid social ethogram? *Veterinary Journal* 181(1), 12–8.

McGreevy, P.D., Docherty, O., Channon, W., Kyrkland, K. and Webster, J. (2017) The use of nosebands in equitation and the merits of an international equestrian welfare and safety committee: a commentary. *Veterinary Journal* 222, 36–40.

McLean, A.N. (2004) Short-term spatial memory in the domestic horse. *Applied Animal Behaviour Science* 85(1–2), 93–105.

McLean, A.N. (2008) Overshadowing: a silver lining to a dark cloud in horse training. *Journal of Applied Animal Welfare Science* 11(3), 236–248.

McLean, A.N. and Christensen, J.W. (2017) The application of learning theory in horse training. *Applied Animal Behaviour Science* 190, 18–27.

Morel, P.C., Bokor, A., Rogers, C.W. and Firth, E.C. (2007) Growth curves from birth to weaning for Thoroughbred foals raised on pasture. *New Zealand Veterinary Journal* 55(6), 319–325.

Murphy, J. and Arkins, S. (2007) Equine learning behaviour. *Behavioural Processes* 76(1), 1–13.

Nazarenko, Y., Westendorf, M.L., Williams, C.A. and Mainelisa, G. (2018) The effects of bedding type in stalls and activity of horses on stall air quality. *Journal of Equine Veterinary Science* 67, 91–98.

Neveux, C., Ferard, M., Dickel, L., Bouet, V., Petit, O. and Valenchon, M. (2016) Classical music reduces acute stress of domestic horses. *Journal of Veterinary Behaviour* 15, 81.

Nicol, C. (1999) Understanding equine stereotypies. *Equine Veterinary Journal (Supplement)* 28, 20–25.

Orlando, L., Ginolhac, A., Zhang, G., Froese, D., Albrechtsen, A. *et al*. (2013) Recalibrating Equus evolution using the genome sequence of an early Middle Pleistocene horse. *Nature* 499(7456), 74–78.

Owen, K.R., Singer, E.R., Clegg, P.D., Ireland, J.L. and Pinchbeck, G.L. (2012) Identification of risk factors for traumatic injury in the general horse population of north-west England, Midlands and North Wales. *Equine Veterinary Journal* 44(2), 143–148.

Padalino, B., Rogers, C.W., Guiver, D., Bridges, J.P. and Riley, C.B. (2018) Risk factors for transport-related problem behaviors in horses: a New Zealand survey. *Animals (Basel)* 8(8), e134.

Parker, M., Redhead, E.S., Goodwin, S.D. and McBride, S.D. (2008) Impaired instrumental choice in crib-biting horses (*Equus caballus*). *Behavioural Brain Research* 191, 137–140.

Pavlov, I.P. (1927) Conditioned reflexes: an investigation of the physiological activity of the cerebral cortex. *Nature* 121(3052), 662–664.

Peters, S.M., Bleijenberg, E.H., van Dierendonck, M.C., van der Harst, J.E. and Spruijt, B.M. (2012) Characterization of anticipatory behaviour in domesticated horses (*Equus caballus*). *Applied Animal Behavioural Science* 138(1-2), 60–69.

Rivera, E., Benjamin, S., Nielsen, B., Shelle, J. and Zanella, A.J. (2002) Behavioral and physiological responses of horses to initial training: the comparison between pastured versus stalled horses. *Applied Animal Behaviour Science* 78(2-4), 235–252.

Rochais, C., Henry, S. and Hausberger, M. (2018) 'Haybags' and 'Slow feeders': testing their impact on horse behaviour and welfare. *Applied Animal Behavioural Science* 198, 52–59.

Rorvang, M.V., Christensen, J.W., Ladewig, J. and McLean, A. (2018) Social learning in horses – fact or fiction? *Frontiers in Veterinary Science* 6(5), 212.

Schubert, M., Jonsson, H., Chang, D., Der Sarkissian, C., Ermini, L. *et al*. (2014) Prehistoric genomes reveal the genetic foundation and cost of horse domestication. *Proceedings of the National Academy of Sciences of the United States of America* 111(52), E5661-E5669.

Seligman, M.E.P. and Maier, S.F. (1967) Failure to escape traumatic shock. *Journal of Experimental Psychology* 74(1), 1–9.

Shalvey, E., McCorry, M. and Hanlon, A. (2019) Exploring the understanding of best practice approaches to common dog behaviour problems by veterinary professionals in Ireland. *Irish Veterinary Journal* 72(1).

Skinner, B.F. (1938) *The Behavior of Organisms: An Experimental Analysis.* Appleton-Century, New York.

Skinner, B.F. (1951) *How to Teach Animals.* Freeman, San Francisco, California.

Stachurska, A., Janczarek, I., Wilk, I. and Kędzierski, W. (2015) Does music influence emotional state in racehorses? *Journal of Equine Veterinary Science* 35(8), 650–656.

Starling, M., McLean, A. and McGreevy, P. (2016) The contribution of equitation science to minimising horse-related risks to humans. *Animals (Basel)* 23.6(3), 15.

Thompson, P.C., Hayek, A.R., Jones, B., Evans, D.L. and McGreevy, P.D. (2014) Number, causes and destinations of horses leaving the Australian Thoroughbred and Standardbred racing industries. *Australian Veterinary Journal* 92(8), 303–311.

Thorndike, E.L. (1898) Animal intelligence: an experimental study of the associative processes in animals. *Psychological Monographs: General and Applied* 2(4), 1–109.

Valenchon, M., Levy, F., Moussu, C. and Lansade, L. (2017) Stress affects instrumental learning based on positive or negative reinforcement in interaction with personality in domestic horses. *PLoS ONE* 12(5).

Voith, V.L. (1986) Principles of learning. *The Veterinary Clinics of North America: Equine Practice* 2(3), 485–506.

Wagner, A.E. (2010) Effects of stress on pain in horses and incorporating pain scales for equine practice. *Veterinary Clinics of North America Equine Practice* 26(3), 481–492.

Warren-Smith, A.K. and McGreevy, P.D. (2008) Preliminary investigations into the ethological relevance of round-pen (round-yard) training of horses. *Journal of Applied Animal Welfare Science* 11(3), 285–298.

Waters, A.J., Nicol, C.J. and French, N.P. (2002) Factors influencing the development of stereotypic and redirected behaviours in young horses: findings of a four year prospective epidemiological study. *Equine Veterinary Journal* 34(6), 572–579.

Werhahn, H., Hessel, E.F., Bachausen, D. and van den Weghe, F.A. (2010) Effects of different bedding materials on the behavior of horses housed in single stalls. *Journal of Equine Veterinary Science* 30(8), 425–431.

Werhahn, H., Hessel, E.F. and van den Weghe, H.F.A. (2012) Competition horses housed in single stalls (ii): effects of free exercise on the behavior in the stable, the behavior during training, and the degree of stress. *Journal of Equine Veterinary Science* 32(1), 22–31.

Wisniewska, M., Janczarek, I., Wilk, I. and Wnuk-Pawlakb, E. (2019) Use of music therapy in aiding the relaxation of geriatric horses. *Journal of Equine Veterinary Science* 78, 89–93.

2 Handling the Horse

Restraining Horses

Handling horses safely on the ground is imperative for all concerned with their daily care, as large, heavy animals with unpredictable natures can easily cause injury. Vets in particular are often injured as the result of equine work, and it is reported that they have little personal or taught knowledge of horse behaviour, compounding the problems they face (Docherty *et al.*, 2017). Restraint of horses is often discussed in the formal education and training of new handlers, and experienced by many in very different circumstances with mixed effects. Restraints are reported to be used commonly in settings where horses need procedures that they may find aversive, such as clipping, dental work and veterinary treatment (Ali *et al.*, 2017). Vets in general experience high rates of injuries, and working with horses they are exposed to fast-moving, unpredictable large animals (Beaver, 2019). Therefore, restraints of all types are sometimes essential in many circumstances with horses, where training alone cannot overcome the pain or distress caused by a procedure.

These restraints can either be physical, such as a particular type of bit or cross-tying (Fig. 2.1), or chemical, and act as a sedative to subdue the horse. Chemical restraints can be administered by any person if they consist of a paste supplied by the vet, but by law only vets are able to inject any category of sedative. Chemical restraints are extremely useful, but sometimes not practical due to the veterinary involvement needed, or in certain procedures such as clipping where they may cause sweating that is contrary to the process of the clip. The most common physical restraints are discussed here, supplemented with evidence from scientific research if it exists.

The Chifney bit, or anti-rearing bit, is a common sight in equine yards, and is often used very frequently where youngstock, Thoroughbreds, or stallions are handled. It is a circular bit and its thin curved bar rests on the tongue, generally also incorporating an inverse port (Fig. 2.2), and the bit has rings to attach to a partial head collar (Fig. 2.3) or a lead rope. The action is similar to a normal bit in that it presses the tongue into the bars of the mouth, but has no joint, therefore the inverted port subjects the tongue to even more pressure against the bars. Even though it is frequently used, there have been reports of this type of bit cutting the horse's tongue due to its shape and thinness (McLean and McGreevy, 2010). The severe downward pressure acts as a 'brake' on the horse that wants to rear, generally stopping it attempting to do so through the application of pain to the lower jaw. The Chifney bit (or a bridle, and sometimes a combination of both) has to be used by law at all UK racecourses when leading the equine competitors, reportedly for safety reasons (British Horseracing Authority, 2019).

The 'twitch' is another regularly used piece of equipment for equine restraint, and has various designs (Fig. 2.4). They are all based on a pinching action, with some having a short length of rope attached to a wooden stick (Fig. 2.5), and others with nutcracker-shaped metal ends. The rope is placed over the horse's upper lip, and is then twisted round and round to tighten on to the lip, leaving a portion of tissue exposed at the very end. The nutcracker metal type is placed around the same area and squeezed tightly to incorporate the same effect. The twitch is thought to action the release of endorphins into the horse's bloodstream, though there is little evidence for this some research has taken place. In an application of the lip twitch for 5 minutes, horses' heart rates dropped significantly; however, if left on for longer than 5 minutes the heart rate considerably increased (Flakoll *et al.*, 2017). This suggests small time periods of application may be useful for restraint, but application of the device beyond that time may cause more distress than previously thought and it was recommended that vets should use chemical restraints for welfare purposes. In other research the same results were seen with the twitch (Ali *et al.*, 2017), and when

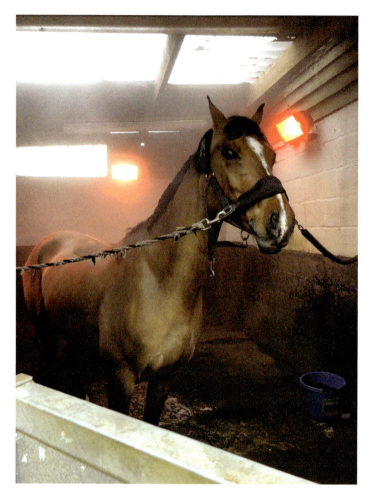

Fig. 2.1. Cross-tying is practised quite frequently as a limited restraint procedure when horses need to stand still in a stable – this horse is receiving infra-red treatment to dry its coat.

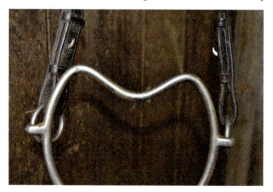

Fig. 2.2. A Chifney bit demonstrating the inverse port designed to put pressure on the tongue and on the bars of the mouth when pulled downwards, such as when the horse rears.

applied for the second time horses showed no aversive reaction to its presentation. However, it was stressed again that the short treatment time should be used, and indeed the researchers commented that they were not endorsing the twitch in place of appropriate techniques using training for unpleasant procedures.

Other restraints have no scientific research to date, and these include the chain shank, or a version named the 'war-bridle'. They consist of a length of chain on the end of a normal rope lead, which is threaded through the lateral rings of the headcollar so that it rests on top of the nasal bone. The horse is then restrained by putting pressure on the chain, so it clamps the nose tightly, causing pain if the horse tries to move. Advice follows that if the horse will still not stand still, the chain can be passed under

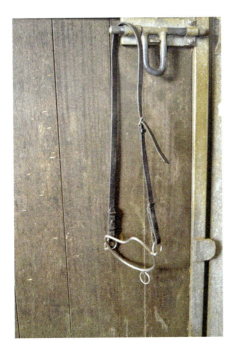

Fig. 2.3. The Chifney is mounted on a partial headcollar, which is used on its own, fastened over another headcollar, or worn in conjunction with a bridle.

the top lip to lie against the upper gum line and tightened here instead. The war-bridle version employs the same equipment, but the chain is placed inside the horse's mouth where the bit would lie, and pressure is applied on the tongue and bars of the mouth. Another version that acts on the same principle is marketed and used across the equine world as a humane method: it uses a system of pulleys and a rope that again lies under the upper lip against the gum line. This is then tightened and clipped on to the headcollar and the horse is restrained by the end of the device. It is possible that no modern research has taken place with these inventions due to ethical concerns of the action of these types of restraint, and indeed requests to carry out the research would probably be refused.

Problems Investigated

Biting

Horses can bite as a natural behavioural conclusion to a warning generally given before the action takes place. The ears pinned back is the most observed communication behaviour (Luz *et al.*, 2015), but the warning they make may not be seen quickly

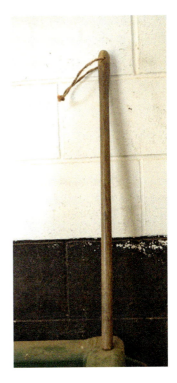

Fig. 2.4. A twitch consisting of a wooden pole with a length of rope attached through the top. The rope is placed over the upper lip of the horse and twisted tight.

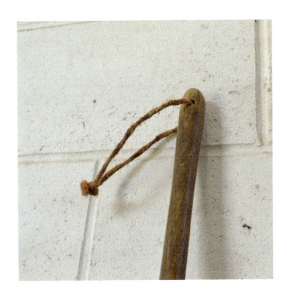

Fig. 2.5. Detail of the top of the twitch illustrating the position of the rope.

enough or could be misinterpreted if handlers are not familiar with the communication of the horse (Fig. 2.6). A quick sideways glance, ears held slightly back, a furled lip – these may be the only sign the horse uses as a warning preceding the biting behaviour. As humans become accustomed to the horse in their care, they will be better able to read these signs and to recognize them in other horses, therefore enabling them to react quickly.

Biting is not always a sign of aggression towards the handler. It could be a redirected behaviour, as previously discussed, and stem from a girth being overtightened, or possible gastric pain (Millares-Ramirez and Le Jeune, 2019). The horse reacts to this pain by biting anything in its way, including its handler, therefore redirecting the behaviour. There

is also some evidence to suggest that horses prone to crib-biting are more likely to show physical sensitivity (Briefer Freymond *et al.*, 2019), so it is possible that this may also be the case for those horses susceptible to developing biting as a problem behaviour. As horses are habit-forming and one-trial learners, biting can quickly manifest as the go-to behaviour when the girth is tightened, whether it causes pain or not. If a horse suddenly starts biting when something different takes place, it is always worth checking to see if there is an underlying pain issue. However, as the biting will probably repeat, even if the pain situation has been resolved, it is useful to be able to stop it.

Horses may also start biting if they are punished, as punishment increases aggression towards the

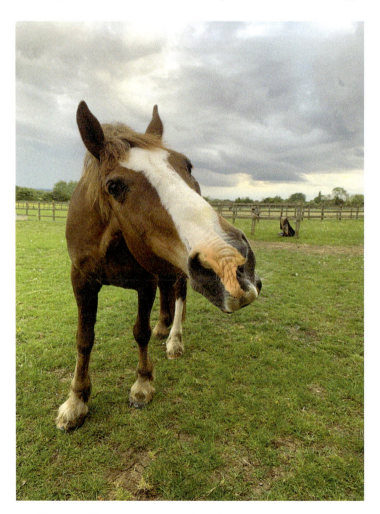

Fig. 2.6. Is this pony reaching out to bite, or just being inquisitive? Handlers need to be able to tell the difference.

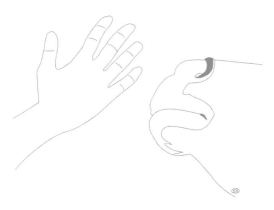

Fig. 2.7. Handlers must never be tempted to hit a horse that bites – punishment will only escalate the behaviour.

handler and reinforces its use as a way to cope with problems (Mills, 1998). Not every horse will do this, but some will react in this way, and a dangerous situation can develop if the punishment continues because the horse has bitten and the handler reacts by hitting the horse again. It is never a good idea to punish a horse: as already discussed, animals will often link the pain to its origin, and because some horses will use aggression as a communication in their natural behaviour it can escalate to them biting the person using punishment (Fig. 2.7). Hitting a horse or using some aversive method may be in danger of creating this situation, so other techniques need to be used to correct this undesirable behaviour.

There is some intriguing evidence for the type of bedding used having an effect on horses and their tendency to bite at or towards their neighbours. It has been reported that horses bedded on straw were less likely to develop aggressive biting as a behaviour (Kwiatkowska-Stenzel et al., 2016). The reason for this might extend to the availability of straw as a food source; therefore the horse is able to spend more of its time in a stable performing the maintenance behaviour of eating and chewing rather than in frustration at being prevented from doing so. This may provide another tool for horsepersons to use with an animal prone to biting, or to use straw if at all possible as a precaution to prevent biting occurring in some cases.

Before developing a plan for the treatment of biting, any pain issue needs to be eliminated first, especially if the biting has developed suddenly. Once this step has been taken, the simple step of ignoring the horse is used. Every time the horse goes to bite, it is ignored, and no reaction is given by the handler at all. Due to behavioural extinction, the horse will

stop the behaviour once it is not getting a reaction, though this may take a long time depending on how ingrained the action is. However, it only needs one reaction by someone to the biting and the schedule of retraining is broken. This is obviously very difficult to police or monitor if the horse has multiple handlers. Horses have excellent memories and if the issue is in origin one of a pain, the animal may never stop biting in certain situations, such as girth tightening. In such cases, the handler needs to appreciate that the situation involves redirected behaviour and must eliminate their feelings of needing to punish the offending horse.

Another method worth trialling consists of using 'differential reinforcement of other behaviour', explained in Chapter 1, and comprising rewarding the horse when the behaviour is not being performed (Fox et al., 2012). This acts to reinforce those periods where biting is not taking place, therefore using positive reinforcement in a slightly different way, without any actual behaviour by the horse but rather an absence of behaviour. The horse is tied up loosely, with the handler standing nearby with a treat reward. When the horse bites, or tries to bite, the handler again ignores it, but the horse is rewarded as soon as it is standing still again it. This enables the horse to learn that biting does not bring a reward, but that not biting, or the absence of biting, does.

The final note on biting involves the sometimes-heard myth that feeding treats leads to this behavioural problem. There is no evidence that this is the case, and although research reports that horses if trained by positive reinforcement with treat rewards might become more likely to search the handler for treats, it does not appear to lead to biting itself. Therefore, those who like to train using treat rewards, and also handlers who wish to use treats for greeting their horse, such as in the field, can have the confidence that biting will generally not happen.

Key points

- Biting can develop from redirected behaviour.
- This could be caused by overtightening a girth, or a pain issue such as gastric problems.
- If a horse is punished by the handler in some situations, it may bite as a reaction to the punishment.
- Try to avoid punishing a horse for biting, as it will worsen the problem.
- Ask everyone who handles the horse to refrain from punishing or shouting at it but just to ignore it.
- Remember that treat rewards will not lead to biting.

Take-home message

Explore redirected behaviour and consider how it may lead to a horse using biting as a tool to avoid an unwanted or unpleasant situation.

Case study

An ex-racehorse was purchased straight from the yard of a trainer by a person experienced in handling horses. Once the horse had been brought home and given time to settle, the first time it was tacked up and its girth tightened it swiftly turned around and bit the handler. Hitting the horse was the first action the handler took, as it seemed to work on the cobs and riding ponies she had trained before. However, in this case the horse lashed out again and bit the handler quite badly. This caused the handler to avoid tacking up the horse without each time restraining it closely and being ready with a whip to punish the horse every time it tried to bite. A call was made to the behaviourist, who came out to visit the horse and watch the litany of girth tightening, biting, punishment and biting again. The rider also mentioned that the horse was becoming

more difficult to control and tried to turn and bite even when being ridden. This was a longstanding problem, and the handler was informed it would take quite a while to correct, if it could be done at all. The problem with pain and redirected behaviour was explained, and the horse was referred to a vet for ulcer inspection. In this case, none of any significance was found, and a diagnosis of redirected behaviour from previous pain was given. The handler and all those who dealt with the horse began to ignore it instead of using punishment, and over the rather long period of 6 months the horse stopped biting altogether.

Striking out

The action of striking out is part of a dangerous behavioural repertoire grouped around the use of the front feet (Fig. 2.8). This is thought to originate from communication in herds, where striking out may be a warning to other horses to keep away or move back (Luz *et al.*, 2015). It is often commented anecdotally that this is a 'dominant' behaviour, used to try to intimidate the handler. However, it is

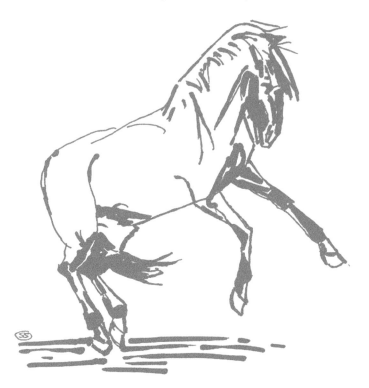

Fig. 2.8. Striking out at a human can be a very dangerous behaviour and needs to be solved before accidents happen.

extremely important to remember that horses do not have a settled herd hierarchy in the wild (Henshall and McGreevy, 2014), or a constant leader, so the action of the handler taking the role of a dominant leader will not necessarily work. There may also be links with the less aggressive behaviour of pawing, though there is currently no evidence that one progresses to the other.

When this behaviour is enacted in the domestic situation, there are several reasons for its origin. It could be linked to a sudden, extremely aversive environment the horse finds itself in. For example, a handler may be rough putting a bridle on and the bit knocks the horse in the teeth – this could cause it to react by striking out as a warning, and as horses are one-trial learners the behaviour could be repeated in stressful situations. This may quickly become a hard-wired behaviour and trialled whenever the horse is handled, not just when the handler approaches with a bridle, but also with the saddle or a rug. It has also been reported as a frustration behaviour (Rochais *et al.*, 2018) when motivation exists for the horse to eat, but it is prevented from doing so. This causes the horse to strike out at whatever is thwarting its behavioural need, and this could indeed be a handler or anyone near the animal. It has also been reported as a frustration response to being asked to stand still (Peters *et al.*, 2012) when motivation exists for it to move, such as herd companions leaving the area.

As the formation of the behaviour against humans probably originates in one-trial learning associated with frustration, the action of training the horse to stop this behaviour can be difficult. The process of positive reinforcement using a treat-based approach does appear to work very well to extinguish this behaviour. Punishment in this situation certainly would not work, as the addition of an aggressive approach with punishment will only serve to heighten the horse's aroused state and possibly also increase the unwanted behaviour. The horse may well associate the punishment to the handler, and its level of aggression may also increase due to this phenomenon. The situation here is somewhat different to others as it is potentially dangerous, so the ability to use learning theory and assess the situation is extremely important for handler safety.

Due to the danger of this behaviour, a strict retraining will need to take place, with all the people involved with the horse informed of exactly what will be happening. In this case the reward process of positive reinforcement could work well, changing the situation to one of appetite response instead of aversive or differential reinforcement of other behaviour as previously discussed. This may need to involve treat-based reward, either through food or voice/scratches, and this judgement needs to be made based on the evidence seen. Timing is crucial here, where the treat must be given when the horse does not react by striking out but ignoring the horse when it does perform this behaviour. This will take time, but the aggressive horse does respond remarkably well when the arousal state is lowered, and it realizes there is no benefit to reacting in this way. Horses do not generally use this behaviour when in a free area; it tends to be displayed when the animal is in a confined space. This could explain the action as being one of inability to get away from the situation it has been placed in, so looking at the environment and possibly increasing turnout and exercise may also benefit the horse.

It is interesting to note that the case study used below does involve a horse developing the behaviour in a field situation; therefore the measures taken to stop it can also surprise the handlers who do not have a knowledge of how the horse processes its environment.

Key points

- Striking out is an aggressive behaviour and can be dangerous.
- It may arise from a simple action such as banging the horse's teeth with the bit.
- There are also links with motivation and prevention of access to food.
- Horses are one-trial learners and could adopt this problem from one incident only.
- Punishment will only aid the level of aggression and cause it to rise.
- A carefully managed retaining of reward and ignoring the behaviour will help to extinguish the behaviour.
- The horse's environment must be considered.

Take-home message

It is worth looking at practices used to tack up/rug up horses and how feeding takes place. The solution can sometimes be found just by changing the environment. Remember, however, that some behaviours are dangerous, and these need to be resolved as soon as they manifest.

Case study

This was an unusual incident where the young horse involved suddenly started striking out in the field when the owner was bringing feed buckets to each horse (the youngster had recently moved into the field for 24 hours a day with a bonded pair). It was winter, and the owner used the well-known method of putting hay in more piles than there are horses to make sure the youngster in this case was getting enough hay. However, when feed was brought into the equation this was a large motivation for the youngster, and it began to strike out at the owner when they approached. The behaviour of all the horses was observed, at feed time and when hay was delivered, to get a clear perspective of what was involved. Due to the inherent danger of this problem, drastic measures were taken and at night the youngster was brought back into a stabled environment, where it received its feed and hay without any distraction from the other horses. This worked extremely well and the horse stopped striking out at the owner almost immediately, without any other training taking place.

This situation illustrates that the problem was quite unusual, but relatively easy to discover what was happening to cause the horse to strike out, and the resolution was also straightforward. It is interesting to note that the striking-out behaviour was directed at the owner bringing the food, rather than at the horses who were creating the event where the youngster felt he had to struggle to obtain his food.

Barging

The problem of barging and pulling when leading is one that has resulted in a plethora of different headcollars (Ijichi *et al.*, 2018) and devices entering the market to attempt to help handlers control their horses more effectively on the ground. It is obvious that this is a serious problem experienced by quite a few owners across disciplines and breeds. The origins are numerous, and as always with behavioural problems it is not necessarily easy to pinpoint the cause. Perhaps the problem in one horse could stem from insufficient training as a foal, or it could be as diverse as a flight incident when a young horse experiences a novel and frightening event. Whatever the cause, barging in this section is

exhibited as an uncontrollable burst of speed, perhaps ending very quickly in the case of barging through a stable door, but also seen by handlers as a lack of concern by the horse for their personal space.

Communication in feral herds does involve amounts of pressure, either tactile or from a distance, whether it is merely with a glance that is enough to cause a less aggressive horse to back away, to a threatening raising of the leg before a kick. Horses will also use the pressure of their bodies to push others away, and this could possibly be the origin of its use against humans, but it is not certain. It is natural for a human to push a horse with pressure, for example to ask it to move over, and perhaps the horse will consequently use it against humans (McGreevy *et al.*, 2009). Possibly, the action of the horse may be just to get away from the frightening situation, and the human being in the way may simply be circumstantial. In the case of barging through stable doors, this may be a reaction to the horse bumping its hip or other sensitive area on the door frame, and then in the future rushing as quickly as possible past the point that caused it pain. This can lead to barging through other entrances, as the horse generalizes the stable door to other gates and openings.

Stopping a horse from barging really lies in retraining basic responses and leading so that the horse responds to the handler when asked to stop or slow down (Fig. 2.9). Barging is generally related to handling or pre-feeding problems (Hockenhull and Creighton, 2012), so returning to foundation training and retraining leading can solve this behavioural problem rather easily. Using learning theory, the horse is retrained to lead correctly and to respond to pressure-release as accurately as possible (Fig. 2.10). This training should be carried out in a safe place, such as a school, and it is important with this type of issue to retrain the horse to respond to a progressively lighter pressure on the headcollar rope. Once the groundwork has been completed, the horse, if trained correctly, will walk through stable doors and other gates with pressure on the headcollar to slow its response. It is possible some horses may trial the barging behaviour again, but with continuous, consistent handling the problem should be alleviated and the behaviour extinguished.

Key points

- Barging is a dangerous problem behaviour and it is always worth retraining.
- Groundwork is the key to solving barging.

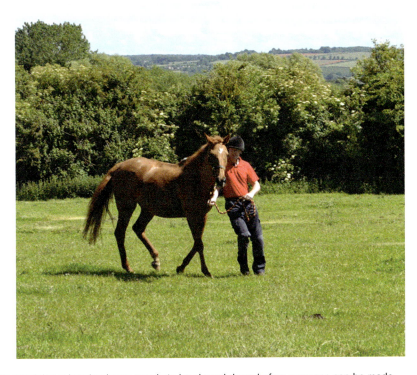

Fig. 2.9. When retraining a barging horse needs to be slowed down before progress can be made.

- Everyone handling the horse must use the same methods until the behaviour is extinguished.
- Be aware, as with all learnt behaviours, that the horse may trial it again in stressful circumstances.

Take-home message

You do not need to resort to buying a specific device to stop the horse barging – try a period of retraining and make sure all handlers are willing to follow the training programme.

Case study

A new pony at a riding stables barged out of its door on the first morning it was being turned out. The handler let go of the pony and it bolted into the yard, causing havoc amongst the riders waiting for lessons. After that event the pony was led everywhere in a bridle, in and out of its stable and to the field and back. The call-out was for something else, but the situation with the pony and the use of the bridle was noticed and help was offered due to the context of the problem. During a booked session the main handler was taught how to use groundwork effectively in a headcollar, and to work with the pony in question in a school until it was retrained to the lighter pressure of the headcollar. The handler progressed to taking the pony around the yard, and finally in and out of its stable. The use of learning theory in the form of groundwork with negative reinforcement enabled even the younger handlers to lead the pony safely, although they were still supervised at all times.

This was an interesting call because the problem was noticed and help offered – handlers at the school were often rushing about trying to get horses ready in time and the additional method of using a bridle for the pony was sometimes forgotten, with dangerous results. It was also a beneficial lesson to learn for the manager of the riding school, in considering timings of lessons and numbers of horses and ponies used to lessen the need for hurrying to

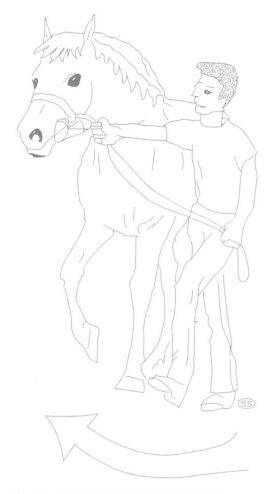

Fig. 2.10. A barging horse will sometimes pull sideways away from the handler, so retraining with leading protocol needs to include the conditioning of lateral movement if this is the case.

meet deadlines. Where cases like these arise, other important procedures may be side-lined or forgotten, but manageable risks cannot be taken when dealing with animals as large as horses. Solving behavioural problems can often lead to much safer environments for humans to work with horses and ponies, particularly when the number of minors who work with these animals is considered.

Leading

Every horse and pony at some point in its training is taught to lead (Fig. 2.11). Problems arise when learning theory is not used effectively by enabling a

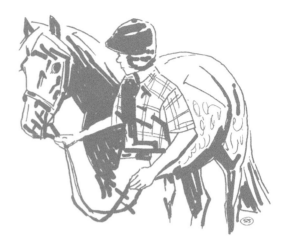

Fig. 2.11. Horses should be trained to lead correctly as part of their basic skill set.

reward to the horse of release of pressure. Horses undergoing leading training with negative reinforcement should always be rewarded with release of pressure once the horse has responded in the correct way, such as stopping when asked or moving off into a walk or a trot, for example by pressure from the lead rope on to the headcollar. Horses generally display learning in the form of classical conditioning, moving when the handler moves, and potentially then ignoring the pressure on the headcollar or not understanding what it means. This can quickly escalate to a horse that will not respond to pressure on the headcollar, as they have had no reward so have not learnt they can remove the pressure by stopping. If this happens, and a horse is motivated to get to its field, or food, or into a stable with hay, it may worsen to a point where the animal pulls the handler in the direction it wants to go – not because of any anthropomorphically perceived misbehaviour but because it has learnt that this is possible.

As leading is such a basic skill for the horse, it should be fully trained before any attempt in further breaking the horse to tack and a rider takes place. However, on busy yards where time is money it can be seriously overlooked and, as with barging, different types of headcollars that increase pressure are used to alleviate the problem. Simply put, retraining a horse to lead correctly encompasses the handler having knowledge of learning theory, and what exactly negative reinforcement is. Domestication has produced many different training methods, but for some unknown reason humans quite often do not align these with the researched psychological techniques of learning theory (McGreevy, 2007). In many cases learning theory is misunderstood, and the action of release of pressure at the correct time is not taken. Therefore, correcting problem leading behaviour involves the horse or pony in question going through a retraining programme, with correct use of negative reinforcement as explained in a previous section. Once this is undertaken, most horses will respond favourably to the retraining, but, as stipulated before with other problems, the handlers involved must all conform to the correct method of pressure-release so that learning can take place.

A horse that bolts when leading is extremely dangerous and can quickly escalate into rearing if headcollars using pressure methods (such as those with metal components and ones that tighten on the nose when pulled) are introduced. The horse may well stop bolting due to the large increase of pressure from one of these devices, but if there is nowhere else to go the horse may react by going up and therefore learning to rear. Rearing is dealt with in a later section; however, it is always best practice to actually retrain the problem before it intensifies into another behaviour such as rearing.

Retraining leading is possibly one of the most interesting things the behaviourist can do, as horses are such individuals with their behaviour. A qualified individual will be able to read the horse's actions and decipher from the way it acts on the lead rope how it will be when it is ridden. When training forward motion, if the horse is very eager to walk forward and learns quickly with just a touch of pressure, the handler can predict that the horse will probably be forward-going under saddle. If the horse is at first reluctant to move forward the opposite is true, and it may be lacking in motivation and possibly also have the label of being a 'lazy' horse to ride. This type of horse is actually either lacking in motivation to move forward (there may be something much more interesting it wants to look at, for example food or companions), or it may be exhibiting conditioning such as learned helplessness by developing a 'hard mouth' or being 'dead to the leg'.

As a basic guide, the horse should be retrained in leading from the very beginning to eliminate any unwanted behaviours. This may include groundwork sessions in a school, and every time the horse is handled the ruling for pressure-release must be adhered to. It is advised to use a bridle if the horse is bolting, but make sure no jabbing or jerking on the bit is carried out. The pressure must start low, then build until the horse moves forward, when the pressure is released straight away. Train the forward movement first, then in the same session ask the horse to stop by using pressure on the lead rope and include backing up where pressure is exerted in reverse until the horse moves (Fig. 2.12). Remember to use shaping, so that any small movement of the horse is rewarded by releasing the pressure, even if it is only at first movement of the body in the correct direction.

Even after only the first session, it is possible the handler will be able to train the horse to stand without moving. Remember that horses will usually just follow the handler, and what is preferable is a horse that only moves when it is asked to do so by light pressure on the lead rope (Fig. 2.13). It is possible to test how much the horse has learnt in the session by attempting to walk away from the horse, without putting pressure on the lead rope, to see if it stands still and does not follow. If the horse attempts to follow, ask it by pressure to move back to where it started, every time, until it will stand still without trying to follow. As the training sessions progress, it is possible the horse can be left anywhere in the working environment and it will stand until asked to move. This of course does depend on environmental stimuli and will rarely work in the horse's own space such as a stable or a paddock.

Once the horse is responding well to these leading sessions, it is possible to start reducing the amount of pressure used until it may only be a light touch on the lead rope. Leading in pairs is also a useful exercise for horses to master (Fig. 2.14). As will be discussed later, any groundwork is replicated once the rider is in the saddle, and this type of groundwork is extremely useful for horses that bolt or are lacking in motivation to move forward away from other horses or further environmental stimuli.

Key points

- Leading must be the foundation for any groundwork, even if it appears unimportant.
- Horses should be trained to stand still when needed, and not to follow the handler but only to move forward with pressure on the lead rope.
- Once leading forward, stopping and reversing are all well trained, start to reduce the amount of pressure needed to the lightest possible.
- If retraining a problem with leading, make sure everyone who handles the horse follows the same protocol.

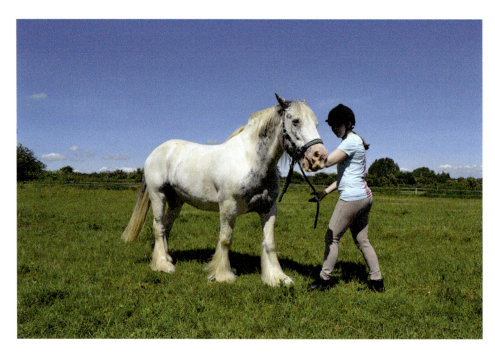

Fig. 2.12. Retraining the reverse movement with pressure on the lead rope to move backwards. Every slight attempt by the horse is shaped with pressure-release.

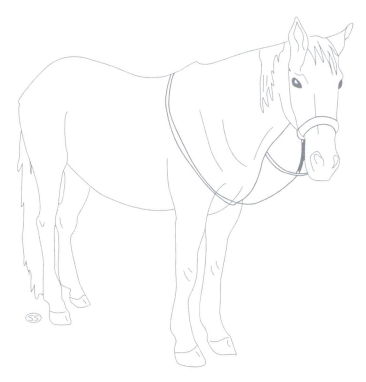

Fig. 2.13. Horses can be trained to stand still without being tied up as part of leading training. Once the horse is only walking forwards and backwards from pressure on the lead rope, then it should stand still if it does not receive a signal to move.

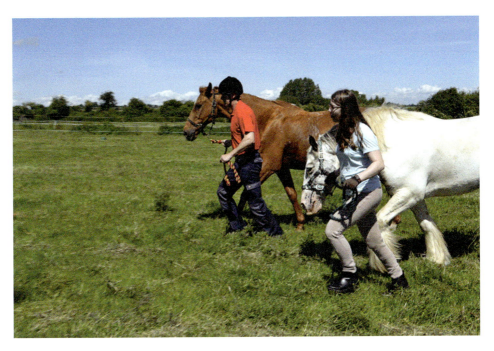

Fig. 2.14. Leading in pairs is also useful for horses to gain experience in working with others.

Take-home message

A well-trained horse will replicate the lessons learned in groundwork once it is ridden, and it is possible to begin retraining behaviours such as bolting by using leading groundwork.

Case studies

A National Hunt racehorse that was very used to following the handlers leading it became problematic when it had to stand still for the vet or farrier, always wanting to have contact with the humans involved. This was solved in the racing yard by carrying out everything needed in the stable – this worked perfectly well until the horse retired from racing and went to another owner who kept it on grass livery without available stabling. There was a small yard to work in, but not a school or arena, so the horse was retrained in the yard with a head-collar and lead rope. The animal in question responded extremely well to the leading training, and within two weeks would stand still in the middle of the yard while the owner carried out other duties. This horse was certainly an exception to the rule and has since proved to be very

responsive to any training it undertakes, particularly in groundwork, and so has been used for student research (Fig. 2.15).

As a contrast case study, a very bulky cob type pony had an extreme case of bolting when being led, to the point that it was becoming dangerous. The owner was using a Chifney, but the pony still tried to run through the bit and managed to pull the reins out of her hands and disappear down the lane. This was an extreme case, and due to this all sessions were strictly limited to the school, where the behaviourist could safely let the pony go if needed.

The cob type pony had a detailed retraining plan, where riding was for the present curtailed as it had begun to pull in canter, which had started to unnerve the owner. The pony was living out at the time and so the owner began the training on the way to the school, which luckily was a short distance, though interestingly the pony never pulled towards the school! Once inside, the owner followed a 20-minute session of leading, backing and standing the horse still, and slowly improvements were made over the period of a month. It was extremely slow progress, but the owner kept to the protocol and soon changed from the bridle to a

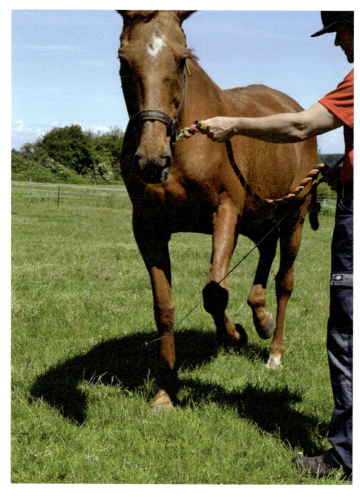

Fig. 2.15. A schooling whip can be also used to signal responses to reverse, so a quick tapping on the most extended foreleg until the horse moves it, along with pressure on the lead rope, may work better with some horses.

head collar when responses were improving. Today the pony is leading correctly, without bolting, but the owner still does groundwork sessions as they feel that without this ongoing training the pony could revert to previous behaviour.

Kicking

The behaviour of kicking is a very common communication tool for the horse when it is with its herd members. In observations they will almost always warn with a raised leg and/or ears back before any kick is attempted, to humans as well as other horses (Fig. 2.16). However, kick injuries are still the most reported reason for fractures in horses, and amount to 43.6% of broken bones seen in domestic herds (Donati *et al.*, 2018). Kicking is also very dangerous for the humans dealing with horses and is the most reported cause of injury (42.5% in total) occurring to owners and riders handling their horses on the ground (van Balen *et al.*, 2019). Those humans who do get kicked are also more likely to have surgery (Kruger *et al.*, 2018) and a higher risk of suffering facial fracture (Islam *et al.*, 2014). These reports really illustrate how hazardous a kicking horse is, and how very important it is for handlers and owners to take the matter seriously.

When horses use kicking behaviour as a threat, it is either in a confined or restrained position where

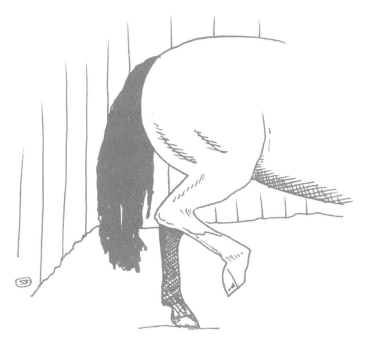

Fig. 2.16. It is useful to be able to recognize when the horse is raising its leg as a threat before kicking – this may be all that handlers see if they react quickly to eliminate or reduce the stimulus the horse is experiencing.

the horse is being asked to perform an action (Fig. 2.17), or when they are being withheld from performing a maintenance behaviour, where the action of kicking is seen as an anticipatory response (Zupan *et al.*, 2019). These situations might range from standing for the vet when a particularly aversive treatment is taking place, to a mare being examined internally, or in the case of anticipatory behaviour if the horse is being prevented by whatever circumstance to be unable to reach, for example, a bucket of feed. The individual singular occasions in which these arise are not usually seen as problematic, as when cornered almost every horse will react in some way to try and escape or prevent the aversive situation. However, if the behaviour is in response to an anticipatory reaction, this may well become hard-wired and may be performed in any pressurized or stressful circumstance.

Retraining this type of problem really resides in treating the horse with sensitivity and understanding, and not putting the animal under any pressure where kicking might be used as a way to escape. This is obviously an extremely difficult procedure, and a horse with this behavioural problem needs to be handled by an expert. It is known that escalating violence to slapping, hitting or even kicking the horse in retaliation will not work, indeed it will act as punishment and increase the horse's level of aggression. Therefore, the handler is only left with careful and thoughtful handling, until the horse is habituated to experiencing only appetitive activities from the human involved. The use of differential reinforcement of other behaviours in retraining may possibly help with stressed horses displaying the behaviour as anticipatory, so that the horse is rewarded when it is not performing the problem behaviour. Relaxing grooming and massage techniques may also help these horses, and as the handling progresses there should be a lessening of hard-wired reaction to aversive situations. However, this behavioural problem can be very difficult to extinguish completely, so this may well remain a horse that will always need to be handled with care.

Key points

- A confirmed 'kicker' is sometimes a dangerous horse to handle and must only be worked on with an experienced horseperson.
- Punishment in any form does not work with these horses, and indeed often actually escalates

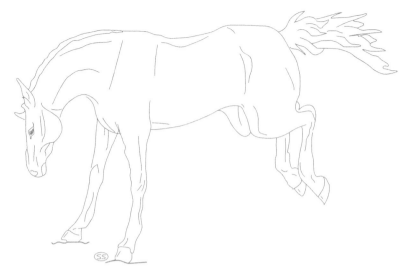

Fig. 2.17. Kicking behaviour when used as a threat can be extremely dangerous.

the problem and incurs more aggression from the horse in question.

- A careful, sensitive approach appears to be the answer, but caution must always be taken even when the behaviour appears to be extinguished.

Take-home message

Horses will generally warn humans before a kick takes place and it is advisable to make sure signs that a horse is stressed or feels under pressure are known. These can include the typical 'ears flat back' posture, but also may include more subtle signs such as a clenched lower jaw and raised neck.

Case study

The horse in this case study was also an ex-race-horse. It had come to the owner through a circuitous route where it had been mistreated by uninformed people not qualified to handle these animals. It was an 11-year-old gelding, quite highly strung, who would kick at people without warning, often when in the field while rugs were being changed. The owner was instructed to find only one other person who would handle the animal, to keep consistency for the horse in its handling. Rug changing was only done once the horse was in the yard, and a system of overshadowing was used to retrain the kicking behaviour. Once basic groundwork

had been completed, leading the horse forwards and backwards a very short distance was used whilst rugging, grooming its belly and other known triggering factors for the kicking behaviour. The horse responded quite quickly, and soon the behaviour was eliminated with the two nominated handlers, though it did on occasion still happen with other people. As time passed this also lessened, to the extent that the horse might still give a warning with a foot lifted in very stressful situations, but did not kick any more.

Door-kicking

The behavioural beginnings of door-kicking are usually associated with appetitive events, such as horses in a yard or barn being fed at various times of the day. For unknown reasons, some horses will wait without any undesirable behaviour being displayed until their food is supplied, whether by bucket or in a delivery system. Others will quickly develop a hard-wired display of door-kicking, whinnying and other displacement behaviours, or during a delayed feeding process by pawing the door (Zupan *et al.*, 2019). Door-kicking in this instance may happen accidentally where the horse kicks the door as the food is being presented and, using its ability for one-trial learning, relates the action of kicking the door to the food finally being supplied. It may also start when the horse is trialling pawing behaviours and hits the door, and then the handler shouts at the horse maybe from the feed room. Many different devices have been used to stop this rather frustrating behaviour, including prickly mats nailed to the lower stable door, the use of an electrical circuit to shock the horse and also usually accompanied by lots of shouting. However, if prevented from kicking at the door, horses can also develop their kicking to using their hind feet on the stable walls (Fig. 2.18). Sometimes horses will be moved into different stables, perhaps closer to the feed room so they get fed first, but these horses will still kick, and the behaviour will never extinguish itself using this method. None of these methods is actually treating the problem behaviour, just either attempting to prevent it by pain or lessening it by moving the horses. It is much more humane to use a retraining solution that works rather than putting into place measures that may affect the welfare of the horses involved.

Handlers also need to consider that the horses in their care will very quickly learn to recognize car engines, or the sound of feet approaching, and that they can distinguish humans when exposed to singular stimuli such as just sight, only smell and no more than hearing (Lampe and Andre, 2012). Horses have extremely complex senses and can react to the cues of sight, hearing and smell by starting door-kicking long before the feed room door is even opened. Of course, as soon as feed-related noises such as buckets and scoops are heard, the horses involved will simply react to a greater extent, and when handlers then shout at them this will only encourage their behaviour. It is also important to remember that horses do not seem to learn by copying each other (Burla *et al.*, 2018; Rorvang *et al.*, 2018): it may be that the only reason there are a number of horses who kick their doors is due to the environment and shared husbandry rather than observational learning.

It is likely that each individual case's origin can never be totally deciphered, but luckily this problem is often one of the easiest to cure, provided that the handlers involved all follow the same procedure. At feeding time, handlers must be very careful not to shout at the horses, but to prepare the feed buckets quietly. Then, when everything is ready, the handler can provide the food to each horse but only presenting that food to the door-kickers when they are not kicking. Opening the door and pushing the bucket through while they kick only positively reinforces the behaviour, in the form of reward for the door-kicking. Any kicking, or whinnying, must be completely

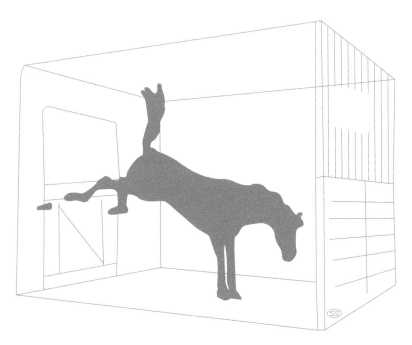

Fig. 2.18. Horses generally kick at their stable doors with their front feet, but kicking in general has also been reported.

ignored. Slowly, over a few days, the horses will stop kicking when they realize that this action does not bring food any more quickly. The motivation to kick is not worth the effort and so it is extinguished. However, it must be noted that every single person dealing with those horses at feeding time must follow the same practice – one shout will reverse the effects of the training and cause the horses to have the reward of attention again.

Key points

- Horses do not copy each other, therefore a stable full of door-kickers is due to the poor environment they are housed in.
- While retraining, everyone involved must follow the same protocol, and avoid the temptation to shout at the horses at feeding time.
- There may well be welfare issues involved if devices that cause pain are used to attempt to stop this behaviour.

Take-home message

When instructing the people at the yard, make sure that the protocol for this retraining is followed exactly – if one person does not follow instructions the learning process will be lost and the horses will revert to door-kicking.

Case study

The experience given here did not involve an actual behaviour consultancy appointment, but was certainly an extremely good example of how quickly horses will stop door-kicking if correct procedures are put in place. Two horses were moved to a new yard, and as the stables closest to the feed room housed the horses that displayed door-kicking behaviour, these two were given stables right at the end of the row. The first morning food was prepared in the feed room to a cacophony of kicking and whinnying, and then carried down the row to the new horses at the end. These two horses had never showed kicking behaviour, and waited for their food to be supplied whilst surrounded by quite a lot of noise. The new owner completely ignored the other horses, knowing how to deal with the problem, and proceeded to feed the new occupants. For the next week, the new owner came early to the yard, quietly fed her own horses and ignored the rest. As the week

progressed, the door-kicking lessened until by the end of six days there was no kicking at all. Interestingly, as soon as the yard manager appeared, while the new horses were being mucked out or groomed, the kicking started again!

The most interesting factor occurred when the new owner took over feeding of all the horses for a week whilst the yard manager was on holiday. The horses were fed in turn, from the feed room and all down the row, and no door-kicking happened at all for the whole week. Were the horses not kicking because they knew this person did not provide food any quicker, or did not shout at them, so there was no motivational point in doing so? It remains unknown, but needless to say the yard manager's return activated the start of the door-kicking, and unfortunately the manager did not want to try out the reconditioning advice offered.

Procedures put in place for larger yards using this advice work very well, but, as before, it is so important that all people involved with the horses do not shout or react towards them if the door-kicking starts. This is certainly not at all easy, especially when people are used to raising their voices when the behaviour occurs, but it is vital for this to happen so that the horses undergo a complete reconditioning process.

Pawing

Pawing can occur in various situations, including at the same time as eating, or expecting feed, being tied up, and when being tacked up ready to hack or school. It is thought to be a behaviour linked to food discovery, such as pawing to uncover grass from snow, or removing the top tangled areas of dead grass from the new shoots below. Owners can easily observe their horses in snowy conditions pawing to get to the grass beneath, and it is this appetitive action that seems to occur when the horse is experiencing frustration involved with inability to get to what it wants. The example of feeding is seen quite commonly across all breeds and types, where the handler places the feed bowl at the horse's feet and while eating the horse paws at the ground or lifts one foot and dangles it above the ground (Fig. 2.19). This situation is not really a problem behaviour, but it can be very difficult to manage when a horse is tied up and pawing the concrete incessantly.

The origin can be estimated and is certainly linked with frustration at the lack of ability to complete

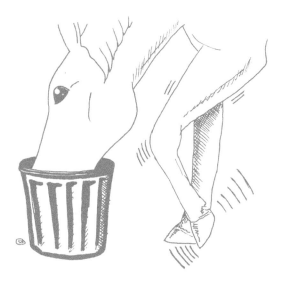

Fig. 2.19. Pawing when being fed is not necessarily a problem behaviour, but it may become so in other circumstances.

tasks where motivation is key. It is classified as a medium-level response to frustration (Young *et al.*, 2012) and therefore an anticipatory behaviour. A horse is taken out of its stable and on most days it would be led out to the field, but when it is to be ridden it is instead tied up in the yard and then paws as a reaction to the powerlessness of its situation (Fig. 2.20). The owner or handler may get frustrated in turn with the perceived lack of patience in the horse; however, it must be understood that horses did not evolve with patience as a key survival factor, like predators, but to react to the moment and keep on the move, either foraging or ensuring their own safety. Predators evolve with the patience for the hunt, whereas prey animals need to react very quickly to escalating situations in their environment.

Solutions to the problem of pawing behaviour when tied up are not easy, due to the levels of frustration that are experienced by the horse. They can be addressed by several methods: there is not a single answer pointing the way to using a particular training method, as it has been found that different techniques appear to work for different horses. However, the technique of positive reinforcement using the differential reinforcement of other behaviour appears to work very well for the majority of animals and reduces the level of frustration, therefore decreasing stress and improving temperament. A reward must be sought for the

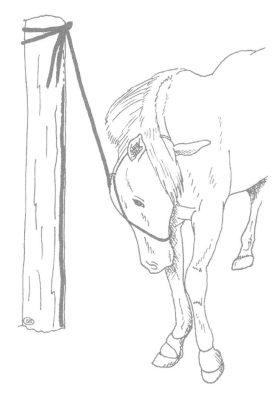

Fig. 2.20. Pawing can become a problem if it is performed when the horse is tied up.

horse in question, and it is generally the owner or handler who has the knowledge for this. After the horse is led out of the stable, it is tied up and then carefully rewarded when it stands still. Every time it paws the ground the horse needs to be ignored, but then rewarded when it is standing still. This is approached through a training session, which needs to be repeated during the week and in conjunction with its usual training.

A particularly mouthy horse, or one that tends to 'mug' people for treats, may need a different approach, such as overshadowing with another, trained behaviour such as target training. Inappropriate behaviours have been seen to fall to nil after target training (Ferguson and Rosales-Ruiz, 2001) so this may be indicated as a training method to trial for pawing. Touching the target could be used as a reward system to overshadow the pawing, with a reward system based on scratching or rubbing the withers or any other appetitive area for that particular horse. Target training is accomplished through operant conditioning, where a horse is presented with a target (which can be anything from a specially designed 'lollipop' stick with a handle and a round area for the animal to touch, to a dandy brush) and rewarded when it touches the objective item with its muzzle. Shaping is used frequently in this training, where even a movement towards the target is rewarded. Due to the inquisitive nature of horses, it is a behaviour that is very quickly and easily learnt and can be developed with the horse touching particular colours or patterns on demand.

Key points

- Horses have not evolved like predators to employ patience amongst their behaviour repertoire.
- There are different methods that can be employed for different horses, depending on temperament and where it is carried out.
- Target training is a useful technique to train a horse, as it can be used in many and various situations.

Take-home message

In various situations horses are expected by humans to display the characteristic of patience. As this is not in their natural behaviour repertoire, owners and handlers must not expect them to comply naturally without training.

Case study

The horse in question was a 7-year-old mare who had been to a horse whisperer for retraining regarding her standing still when tied up. Once the horse had returned home the owner found that she would stay tied up without breaking away but would regularly paw at the ground when being groomed or shod. The horse was visited when the farrier came, and it was clear that the situation was very frustrating for the owner. After some observation of the young mare it was decided that the quickest method possible would be best, as quite clearly the farrier was in some danger: she pawed at the ground totally ignoring where he was positioned. It was so violent that it almost seemed to be a fear response, and the worry was that it would extend to when she was being tacked up in her stable. It would have been interesting to find out what training the horse whisperer had undertaken, but unfortunately for other reasons contact was not possible.

The owner was given a programme of retraining that included very short sessions of standing tied up before being released and walked around the yard, as it was possible the horse had suffered some trauma in her previous training to stand still. The horse was rewarded by lots of scratching whilst stood still, and sooner than expected the mare began to respond to the careful treatment.

Standing still

The behavioural problems associated with a horse not standing still originate from the same set of circumstances where horses, as prey animals, do not understand patience in their behavioural repertoire. If left in an open space such as a school, horses will naturally gravitate towards the exit, even when they have a rider who is not giving them any signals (Burke and Whishaw, 2020). When they move in those circumstances, they walk in looping movements to explore the area, and keep returning to the exit on each loop. Even horses who are never turned out and live in confinement in stables show rapid habituation to free movement once released into a paddock (Le Simple *et al.*, 2020). Therefore, standing still is a learnt behaviour, ideally taught with very early handling skills in foundation training, and if done carefully there should be no problem. However, certain situations such as herd members being led past, or loud noises in the yard, can cause horses to break away from their position.

It is useful to note that most horses in the UK are tied up with their lead ropes attached to a headcollar fastened correctly (Fig. 2.21). This rope is not generally tied straight to the securing point (usually a metal ring, or something convenient like a gate) but to a length of baler twine, readily available from hay or haylage bales and utilized extensively for all sorts of issues in the average equine yard. It is not considered good husbandry to tie the horse straight to the securing point, due to the possibility that the horse might try to break away and be unable to do so, therefore causing a very dangerous situation where the animal may feel trapped and even injure itself. Some horses learn that they can break away if they want to, trained by accident with operant conditioning – the horse pulls and gets the reward of freedom (Fig. 2.22). Once this has become a learnt behaviour, horses will use it in any situation where they may feel threatened or want to pursue their motivational needs to join herd members, or search for food.

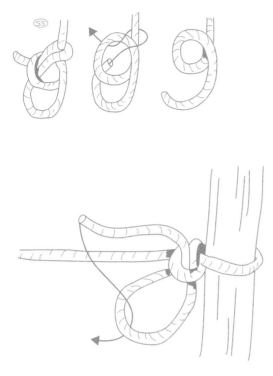

Fig. 2.21. A safety knot for use in tying a lead rope to a piece of baler twine (in this case it is seen tied to a post for clarity).

Problems with standing still may originate from this learnt behaviour, but can be solved most of the time by using a method to overcome the horse's ability to escape without placing it under undue stress of entrapment with the application of a lunge line. At this point it is important to mention that shouting and punishing the horse (as noted before) will only serve to escalate the problem and reinforce any flight behaviours that exist. It is also imperative the horse has had some groundwork training in leading and standing still. Keep any handlers acting calmly around the horse, and make sure the area around the securing point is not crowded or confined, such as in a stable. Using a lunge line as the lead rope, thread it through the ring (Fig. 2.23) or other securing point and then ask the horse to stand. Rewards such as treats if appropriate or scratching/calm words will help at this time. Do not thread the lunge line through baler twine, as the line will need to slip easily. If the horse tries to break away, let it move by allowing the lunge line to run as the horse backs off. At this point ask the horse with slight pressure to stop, and make sure all pressure is removed once it does stop. As soon as the horse stands still, quietly ask it to move back to the original position with minimum pressure.

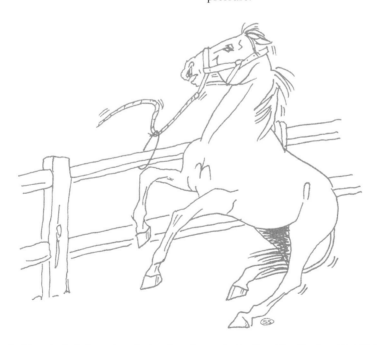

Fig. 2.22. A horse that breaks its tether when tied up is a danger to itself and to other horses and humans if it is loose on the yard.

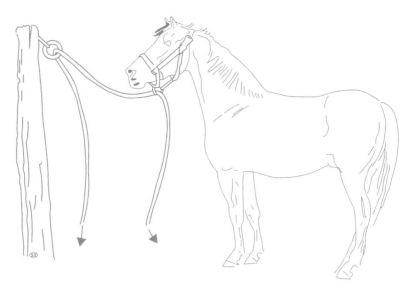

Fig. 2.23. Using a lunge line to retrain a horse that breaks away from its tether – the horse learns that it cannot get away but during training is still able to alleviate its motivation to move.

This method is repeated in every training session, making the procedure as calm as possible and using the leading practice of reversing the horse back into position if needed and applying as little pressure as possible. Each horse, and its past experience, is obviously very different, but this method appears to work rather well and also keeps the situation calm and with minimum stress. If problems do occur, such as the horse backing off very quickly as it trials breaking the string, the handler must apply the method very promptly, making sure there is no pressure on the horse's headcollar, as this appears to be the trigger for the pulling-back behaviour. Once the trigger is removed, and there is no prospect of feeling trapped, this method using a combination of negative and positive reinforcement tends to work extremely well.

Key points

- Do not allow the situation to escalate where the horse is made to feel even more trapped and unable to follow its motivation to escape.
- Use the lunge line carefully – to perfect the technique it is quite a good idea to practise this method with a person on the end of the lunge line instead of a horse.
- Never tie the horse so it cannot break away (see case study) – this is extremely dangerous.

Take-home message

Horses are large animals and if they are put into a position where they feel cornered or trapped it is not unusual for the calmest of characters to display the only behaviours left to them – to kick out, rear up or otherwise try to fight their way out of the situation.

Case study

A pony was referred by the veterinary surgery with the problem of breaking away from its securing point numerous times and then receiving retraining. However, the method of tying it up with a chain to a post had been used, which had caused trauma to its neck. This had compounded the problem, and in this case an adult handler was asked to help with the pony. As soon as pressure was removed from the animal it responded very well to the lunge line method, and within a few days was standing calmly for its young owner. It is possible the intense trauma it suffered was so far removed from the retraining method that it did not link the two. However, as with most behavioural problems and solutions, it is never really revealed what has actually happened except under the guise of learning theory providing a useable resolution.

Catching

Catching is probably one of the most common behavioural problems horsepersons face and refers to the horse or pony being turned out into a paddock or field and then refusing to be caught. There appears to be a gap in research with catching, as some horses will always come to the owner's or handler's call with no training at all, whereas others will only approach if they can see a food bucket. There are even comments regarding the need for eye-to-eye contact to catch horses successfully, though research suggests this is not the case (Verrill and McDonnell, 2008). There are plenty of anecdotal comments from handlers regarding horses not coming near if they are carrying a headcollar, or are wearing certain clothes, or even at varying times of the day. An example given by an owner was that they could catch their horse easily if it was twilight, or beginning to get dark, whereas at any other time the horse was nowhere near as cooperative. There is very little evidence to suggest horses can link events in this manner, i.e. realizing that approaching darkness means they will not be asked to work; however, research needs to be expanded to discover more about this type of learning in horses (Brubaker and Udell, 2016).

Freedom is obviously very important to the horse as a prey animal, and its natural behaviour is centred on unfettered movement and feeding (Fig. 2.24). A horse restricted to a stable is reliant on the handler for its feed and exercise, and situations where handlers feel their horse is 'happy' to come in are probably due to appetitive motivation and not to shelter from inclement weather. Even though horses do not appear to have routines in herd situations, they quickly learn to recognize the signs of coming in;

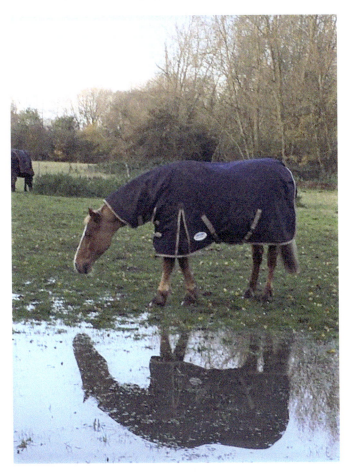

Fig. 2.24. Even in wet weather horses tend to prefer to be outside.

for example, the handler arriving on the yard, approaching darkness and the temptation of a cereal-based food reward. The coming-in ritual is classically conditioned without the handler realizing it, and problems with catching tend to happen when the horse is at grass in the spring/summer/autumn months and not regularly spending the night (or day, if it is hot) in their stable (Fig. 2.25). Horses that are field-kept have no routine of coming in, so potentially every time they are caught they may work. However, as stated, there is no research currently to confirm this possibility.

Nevertheless, a cohort of horses out on grass does present the most problems to their handlers in being caught, and it can be exceedingly frustrating when handlers have an allotted period of time to catch, groom and tack up their horse for exercise. Those who have spent hours chasing their horse around a field only to give up in desperation can bear witness to this circumstance. Solving the problem is not necessarily easy, as there is so much motivation for a horse to stay at grass – freedom, food and possibly also companionship, as already

mentioned. Handlers will often try to tempt the animal with a bucket of feed and make this the motivation for catching them, which can work very well but can be challenging if there are other horses in the field. There are human safety issues that need to be discussed when handling a group of horses kept together (Hartmann *et al.*, 2017), and often communication is warranted amongst livery owners in these circumstances. The uncompromising horse, whose motivation is very much food and freedom, will appear to be a very stubborn personality, but as it is incorrect to categorize a horse as such, other methods must be sought (Fig. 2.26).

It must be remembered the horse has incessant curiosity as part of its behavioural repertoire and this trait can be incorporated into training. In solving the catching problem, the starting advice would include leaving a 'field-safe' headcollar on the horse, to make catching easier, and perhaps a very short length of rope (Fig. 2.27). The approach to the horse then needs to be in a leisurely manner, as horses tend to move slower and at a lesser distance from the handler when they approach slowly (Birke *et al.*, 2011), so if

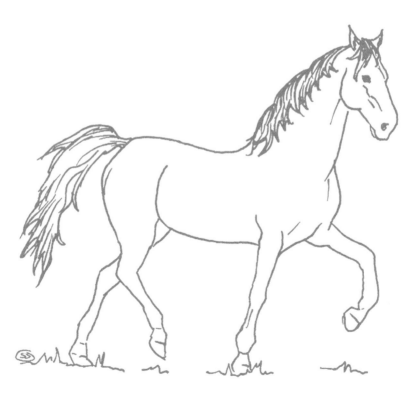

Fig. 2.25. Freedom to graze and move around is a natural maintenance behaviour for a horse – it is not surprising if they protest at being caught.

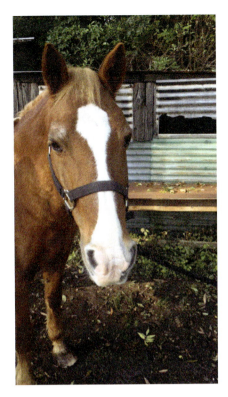

Fig. 2.26. A simple headcollar worn by a pony can help with catching.

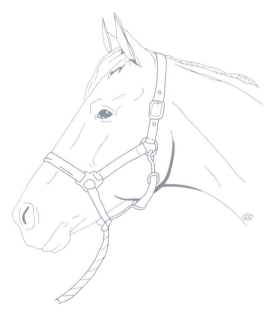

Fig. 2.27. A short length of rope attached to a headcollar may help with catching a field-kept horse.

approached calmly they will not move away as far or as quickly. Once this is in place the first method to try would be positive reinforcement, where a food bucket used as a reward is offered to the horse, and no actual catching is trialled until the animal has lost some of its natural suspicion. Each time, the handler should make a distinctive noise, such as a whistle or calling the horse's name, to condition the sound with the food reward. It is also useful to exploit the horse's colour vision: the colours yellow and blue are most striking, so a feed bucket in a bright yellow can act as a visual cue (Paul and Stevens, 2020). Most horses will respond to a food reward very well, although it is up to the handler to decide the most appetitive treat for the season, for example cereal in the summer when fresh grass is at a premium. Catching up the horse with this method would involve at first a short grooming session, making everything very appetitive for the animal, and releasing quite quickly back into its field. This would be repeated until exercise is included, again perhaps designing more attractive sessions such as a hack with herd companions. Slowly the horse will begin to lose its connection with catching being aversive, although it does appear to be the set default for a certain number of horses. The other method that has proved useful also relies on the horse's natural curiosity and is explained in detail in the case study below.

Key points

- Handlers must remember that horses are not trying to be awkward about catching, even though it may seem like it – the truth is they are fulfilling their motivational needs far more completely by being free in a field with ample food.
- It can be helpful to leave a field-safe headcollar with a short length of rope on a horse that is hard to catch.
- Never chase a horse or pin it in a corner – it may be vital when there is a desperate need to catch the animal, but used on a regular basis it could put the horse into a situation where it feels trapped and needs to strike out if it cannot escape.

Take-home message

Patience, of the human kind, is needed in these cases, and owners and handlers need to remember that if the horse's overriding motivation is for freedom even a tasty full feed bucket will not suffice to bring them in.

Case study

A gelding that had been purchased quite quickly from a dealer on video sale had come from Ireland in a shipment with other showjumpers and its scope was such that the new owner did not overly worry about any behavioural issues with handling, relying on their experience to overcome anything that occurred. A call was placed when it was discovered the horse was almost impossible to catch: the new owner could only herd it into a corner, which obviously was far from ideal. Stabling the horse for 24 hours a day was an option, but not ideal for management of temperament or behavioural issues. On arrival to the call-out the horse had been outside for a few hours and the owner demonstrated the issue very clearly. The gelding would let the owner approach it, but as soon as they became close enough to grab the rope it would trot off out of reach. Even a feed bucket was not enough motivation to be caught, so another method had to be used.

While the horse was grazing, the behaviourist entered the field and walked around the field completely ignoring it, pretending to inspect the fence and ground. Because of its natural curiosity, the horse started to watch the person, who still ignored the animal and carried on walking around. After about half an hour the horse started approaching the person and following them across the field. The crucial part of the exercise had begun, where the horse is still ignored, until eventually the handler turns around and there is usually no problem in catching the horse. It can be more difficult at the beginning for the owner, or whoever the horse is used to, but this method needs patience and will work eventually.

In this case study the horse was far easier to catch after the retraining, though the owner did need to employ the ignoring method a few times and always had to let the horse approach them. One method that the owner also exploited was to use the same yellow-coloured feed bowl and to call the horse's name. One side-effect was that, after the feed bowl conditioning, the horse was always attracted to yellow and proved very interested in grit bins at the side of the road and builders' buckets.

Separation anxiety

Horses and ponies can appear to suffer in some way from this human mental condition, as owners who have seen their horses canter up and down a fence line desperate to get to other herd members. The worst ones even leave tracks along the fence (Fig. 2.28) and

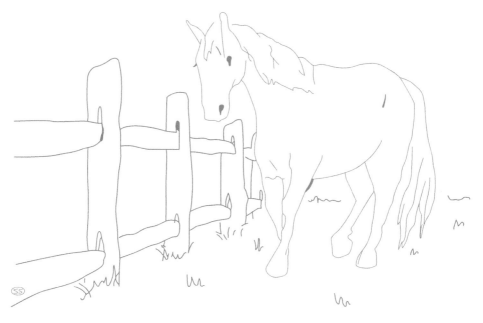

Fig. 2.28. Separation anxiety may be observed in horses walking or trotting along the perimeter of a fence, sometimes frequently enough to wear a path through the grass.

if able will jump out or run straight through electric tape, affording a real problem for owners and handlers to cope with. In evolutionary terms the horse suffering from separation anxiety is only demonstrating its natural behavioural need for companionship. For prey animals there is certainly safety in numbers and they have evolved to possess this motivation, for some to the extreme. Also, as prey animals living in a herd structure, horses crave social interaction and communication with others (Reid *et al.*, 2017).

There are anecdotal reports of pair-bond relationships in horses (Fig. 2.29), and for the owner this might prove very problematic when one horse needs to be separated from the other for whatever reason. Horses may demonstrate increased movement and vocal calling when separated from their favoured partners, and this can raise stress levels and also the risk of injury (Collyer and Wilson, 2016). Pair-bonding can take different forms; for example, one horse may not really be too concerned about coming in away from the other if they are ridden very soon after being separated. They may show no behavioural issues at all, whereas another individual may not be able to be ridden without the other being present. The owner dealing with this pair-bond will probably know the horses very well, and what their limits are, and can take advantage of this knowledge to organize them accordingly. This

is not so easy when horses are competing or must be separated if one becomes ill, so it is useful to have the anxiety over separation controlled as much as is possible in case this happens.

However, horses are individuals, and some appear unconcerned if they are kept on their own or are separated from herd members. Indeed, research has reported that horses who appear to cope better with separation may have had little interference from humans when they were born and immediately after (Henry *et al.*, 2009). It is useful to remember that it is possible their heart rates or cortisol levels are raised, indicating stress without necessarily showing behaviours that humans would equate with separation. Due to this, it is never advised to keep horses or ponies alone without companionship. With evolution as a mitigating factor, it can be seen that solving the problem of separation anxiety is rarely easy. If horses need to be separated it is possible that measures need to be taken such as making sure fences are high enough not to jump, or electric tape is secure, so that the animal cannot leave the field. This is far from ideal, and it is suggested that prevention may be the best method of handling this mental condition. Keeping horses in groups of more than three where horses are routinely removed may stop pair-bonding taking place. Nevertheless, horses are very

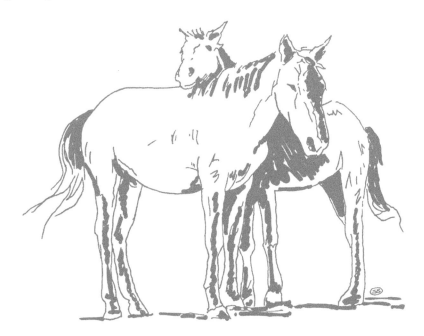

Fig. 2.29. Pair-bonds form between horses kept in groups or sometimes between two individuals kept together.

Handling the Horse

tactile animals and certainly seem to prefer individual companions over others (Fig. 2.30).

For those owners who have no choice but to keep two horses together, there is no quick or straightforward solution in retraining using learning theory, as the advantages of horses having this close companionship is extremely beneficial for their mental and physical health (Fig. 2.31). With these partnerships the way forward to having some control uses desensitization, and again patience is the key. One horse is separated from the other, but only for a very short time before being placed back into the field. This is repeated with both animals, and then the time separated is lengthened very slowly as the two individuals begin to learn that their companion will be returning. Appetitive reinforcers can be used at these times and either feeding or hacking with others may work to distract the separated horse from its companion. The solution in these cases will probably never be fully resolved, but the stress can be lessened to a certain degree by using this slow approach. At the other end of the scale, when one horse is either sold or must be put to sleep, it is very advisable that other horses are on hand ready to be turned out with the remaining individual immediately. Also, if one horse is to be put to sleep, anecdotal evidence from vets appears to be to let the surviving horse investigate its dead companion afterwards. However, other anecdotal reports suggest this could be very traumatic for both the remaining horse and the owner.

Key points

- Keeping horses and ponies on their own is not advised, due to their long evolutionary history of existing as herd animals.
- Pair-bonds do develop between horses and these need to be handled with care, as potentially they are mentally and physically very beneficial for the horses involved.
- More research is needed to investigate the phenomenon of separation anxiety in horses.

Take-home message

Horses live in herds and prefer company of their own kind. When separated from others they will naturally feel more threatened, though some may not show any signs of feeling this way. It is very

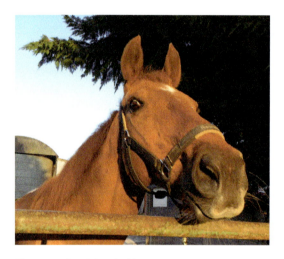

Fig. 2.30. A pair-bonded horse showing signs of anxiety looking out for its companion (white sclera showing in eye, ears pointing forward).

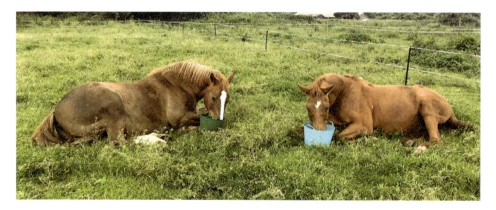

Fig. 2.31. Pair-bonded geldings enjoying breakfast together.

important to make sure horses have a companion of their own species to ensure their mental health.

Case study

Two pair-bonded mares (with different owners) who shared the same field posed no problem initially as they were ridden or led out together and so were never left alone. The problem of separation began when one of the ponies needed to be separated from the other due to developing laminitis. A humane muzzle was trialled at first, but the pony did not keep it on and the situation became life-threatening, so help was sought. The ponies were observed and a method of fencing was introduced so they could still groom each other over the fence, which appeared to work very well. Desensitization sessions were also introduced, which helped the whole situation to be less stressful for each individual, although the owners were very unwilling to test the relationship by riding one of the ponies out, which in this case was very understandable.

Unfortunately, this case study did not end well, as one pony developed an incurable arthritic condition where it progressed past paddock lameness and became uncomfortable in its daily life. The owner of this pony had no choice but to have the pony put to sleep, and advised the other owner of the date and the recommendation from their vet to have another pony in place to move in. Due to unknown circumstances, when the pony was put to sleep no other animal was available, and the pony left on its own displayed very real signs of stress, calling and galloping around. It was reported later that the pony had been found dead in its field about two weeks after the incident and on post-mortem nothing was found to indicate why it had died.

Picking up feet

Horses are generally trained at an early age to pick up their feet for inspection, trimming and/or shoeing. Problems can begin if the farrier hammers in a nail incorrectly and causes pain, or the horse develops an injury or perhaps disease in the foot and it needs to be picked up on a regular basis for treatment, which may be painful. Anecdotally, horses have been reported to develop real fears to lifting their feet if a poultice has had to be applied regularly, as standing on three legs can be quite a difficult feat for young, unbalanced horses or elderly horses with other health problems. As the horse has

tremendous power in its kicking ability, this is a serious problem if the animal is reacting strongly to the attempts made to pick up its feet. The other issue rarely considered is the health and safety of the person involved regarding spinal and back injuries when holding a hoof that the horse is trying to snatch out of their grasp. When handlers were examined for their posture, 88% were not picking up hooves with the best interests of their own health (Lansade et al., 2019), so this must be considered when any retraining is taking place. However, horses will rarely acquire difficulties with picking up feet unless pain is involved to some extent, though as with all behavioural problems the source is not necessarily clear.

In foundation training it is beneficial to use a couple of techniques simultaneously when teaching the horse to pick up its feet. A tap on the back of the lower leg with a command such as 'hup' reinforces the behaviour and enables the handler to use either voice or a touch in the future. It is up to personal taste (Fig. 2.32) but the important aspect is that the horse offers its foot when asked either by voice or by touch or a combination of both. When training using these methods, it is usually beneficial to start with the front feet, as a young horse may feel threatened if the hind feet are picked up first, and it is safer for the handler. The youngster should be very used to handling and grooming, so will learn very quickly to lift its foot on command, perhaps with the addition of reward such as a scratch once the foot is lifted. Progressively the foot is held for longer periods of time, and if the horse's future is to be shod the hoof can be gradually knocked to simulate the farrier's hammer. Another note of interest when training is to make sure the foot is not dropped suddenly but the horse is allowed to lower the foot to the floor naturally to avoid snatching developing when the horse suffers pain if it is just released quickly.

Once trained, the horse will be willing to lift each foot in turn for whatever procedure is taking place, and for those horses that develop a fear of lifting their feet for whatever reason the same techniques are put in place. Clearly, each situation will be different, and with some very fearful horses great care must be taken and handlers should wear hard hats and other personal protection equipment. The training area must be quiet, the number of handlers should be kept to a minimum, and no force should ever be used to pull the foot up off the ground. As with other problems involving a

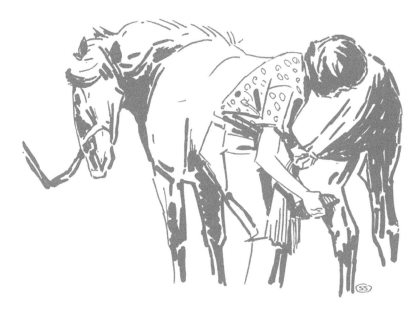

Fig. 2.32. Training horses to pick up their hind feet may involve at first brushing gently around the hind legs to desensitize them.

possible precursor of pain, it is best to be quiet and non-confrontational and try to provide a stress-free environment for the horse to relearn that it can pick up its feet safely without pain or distress. There may be a need for the operant conditioning to be positively reinforced with a motivational reward, such as a treat, and the handler needs to use a voice command and/or a tap on the lower leg at the same time so the horse connects the two, enabling classical conditioning. If the horse has shown an extreme reaction, it is also important to consider shaping, so every slight attempt at lifting the foot is rewarded carefully by the handler. The horse may also need pre-training in the form of desensitization if it kicks out at any attempt to lift its foot, and this can be provided by beginning with grooming the leg and progressing to asking the horse to lift it. In severe cases this may take quite a while, sometimes days, so it is best to deal with foot-lifting problems as soon as possible to avoid any situation where the horse's feet cannot be maintained correctly (Fig. 2.33).

Key points

- A horse that develops problems with picking up its feet must have retraining arranged as soon as

is possible, due to the crucial need of regular horse foot care.
- A cautious and quiet environment must be employed in retraining if the horse has any tendency to kick.
- Shaping is an excellent method to use in these cases, as is a preliminary training period involving desensitization of the lower legs.

Take-home message

Training for picking up feet needs to be one of the very earliest behaviours to teach in the young horse. If horses are taught to lift feet in a certain order, they will become classically conditioned to lift them in that order and be ready to lift the next one once the previous foot has been lowered to the ground.

Case study

A horse was brought to the attention of the behaviourist several years ago in an almost implausible scenario where it was deemed impossible to shoe the horse without a general anaesthetic. Incredibly it was anaesthetized three times a year for the shoeing procedure to be carried out, as no training procedure trialled so far had worked and the owner had decided anaesthesia was the safest

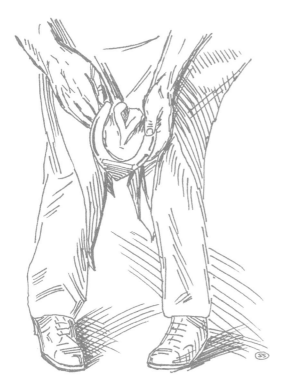

Fig. 2.33. To ensure that regular hoof care can take place, it is essential for horses to be comfortable when lifting their feet.

method to use for this horse. It must be noted that the hind feet were able to be shod – the problem was only with the front feet. The horse was visited when it had just undergone removal of all its shoes to aid the retraining and was observed when asked to lift its feet, which was attempted with a rope tied to the front leg above the knee, then slipped down the leg towards the hoof. Immediately the problem became apparent: the horse was terrified of any contact with its lower leg, becoming extremely dangerous when anything was tried out. The rope trick had worked for a while, but any sort of restraining device can cause problems in a prey animal whose only option, when cornered and unable to flee, will be to try to fight back.

Understandably this was a very deep-seated problem, and the outcome was not at all possible to predict. However, a programme of retraining was agreed with the desperate owner and took place over several weeks. The first exercise was to re-educate the horse in understanding that humans presented no cause for alarm when they approached

any area near its lower legs. Using desensitization, grooming became the tool for training, with a soft brush used to stroke the horse all over its body, and occasionally moving to the top of its legs. The horse was fine with brushing above the knee, so this was accepted as the natural limit of tolerance and brushing below the knee became the target area. The owner took her time, and slowly brush strokes could be applied past this target point, but every time the horse moved or gave signs of stress the brush was moved higher. After a great deal of patience, the owner could brush around the coronet bands on both front feet without a reaction.

Over the next few weeks, foundation training came into play, with brushing changing slowly to tapping and then asking for the foot to be lifted. If the owner moved quietly, and read the horse correctly, they would take the process a step back, progressing to the stage where the stress levels reduced again as and when needed. Gradually the process was repeated on both front feet, and then rapidly the training began to succeed as the horse became more and more relaxed. The owner was soon lifting the feet and could engage a trimmer who was willing to begin to work slowly on the hooves as the horse recovered. It is pertinent at this point to explain that the horse was at a riding/livery stables, and the owner had suffered plenty of negative feedback from others about the treatment of the horse, which was not at all easy for the owner to cope with. Nevertheless, the owner wanted to give the horse the best chance of avoiding being put to sleep and with their patience and dedication they succeeded in this most peculiar case.

References

Ali, A.B.A., Gutwein, K.L. and Heleski, C.R. (2017) Assessing the influence of upper lip twitching in naïve horses during an aversive husbandry procedure (ear clipping). *Journal of Veterinary Behavior* 21, 20–25.

Beaver, B. (2019) *Equine Behavioural Medicine.* Academic Press, London.

Birke, L., Hockenhull, J., Creighton, E., Pinno, L., Mee, J. and Mills, D. (2011) Horses' responses to variation in human approach. *Applied Animal Behaviour Science* 134(1–2), 56–63.

Briefer Freymond, S., Bardou, D., Beuret, S., Bachmann, I., Zuberbuhler, K. and Briefer, E.F. (2019) Elevated sensitivity to tactile stimuli in stereotypic horses. *Frontiers in Veterinary Science* 6, 162.

British Horseracing Authority (2019) *Requirements before mounting.* Available at: http://rules.britishhorseracing.

com/#!/book/34/chapter/s3175-preparing-for-the-race/content?section=s3192-requirements-before-mounting&keyword=chifney (accessed 26 February 2020).

Brubaker, L. and Udell, M.A.R. (2016) Cognition and learning in horses (*Equus caballus*): what we know and why we should ask more. *Behavioural Processes* 126, 121–131.

Burke, C.J. and Whishaw, Q. (2020) Sniff, look and loop excursions as the unit of 'exploration' in the horse (*Equus ferus caballus*) when free or under saddle in an equestrian arena. *Behavioural Processes* 173, e104065.

Burla, J.B., Siegwart, J. and Nawroth, C. (2018) Human demonstration does not facilitate the performance of horses (*Equus caballus*) in a spatial problem-solving task. *Animals (Basel)* 8(6), e96.

Collyer, P.B. and Wilson, H.S. (2016) Does a commercial pheromone application reduce separation anxiety in separated horse pairs? *Journal of Veterinary Behavior* 15, 94.

Docherty, O., McGreevy, P.D. and Parsons, G. (2017) The importance of learning theory and equitation science to the veterinarian. *Applied Animal Behavioural Science* 190, 111–122.

Donati, B., Furst, A.E., Hassig, M. and Jackson, M.A. (2018) Epidemiology of fractures: the rôle of kick injuries in equine fractures. *Equine Veterinary Journal* 50(5), 580–586.

Ferguson, D.L. and Rosales-Ruiz, J. (2001) Loading the problem loader: the effects of target training and shaping on trailer-loading behaviour of horses. *Journal of Applied Behaviour Analysis* 34(4), 409–423.

Flakoll, B., Ali, A.B. and Saab, C.Y. (2017) Twitching in veterinary procedures: how does this technique subdue horses? *Journal of Veterinary Behavior* 18, 23–28.

Fox, A.E., Bailey, S.R., Hall, E.G. and St Peter, C.C. (2012) Reduction of biting and chewing of horses using differential reinforcement of other behavior. *Behavioural Processes* 91(1), 125–128.

Hartmann, E., Christensen, J.W. and McGreevy, P.D. (2017) Dominance and leadership: useful concepts in human-horse interactions? *Journal of Equine Veterinary Science* 52, 1–9.

Henry, S., Richard-Yris, M.-A., Tordjman, S. and Hausberger, M. (2009) Neonatal handling affects durably bonding and social development. *PLoS ONE* 4(4), e5216.

Henshall, C. and McGreevy, P. (2014) The role of ethology in round pen horse training – a review. *Applied Animal Behavioural Science* 155, 1–11.

Hockenhull, J. and Creighton, J. (2012) The strengths of statistical techniques in identifying patterns underlying apparently random behavioral problems in horses. *Journal of Veterinary Behavior* 7(5), 305–310.

Ijichi, C., Tunstall, S., Putt, E. and Squibb, K. (2018) Dually noted: the effects of a pressure headcollar on compliance, discomfort and stress in horses during handling. *Applied Animal Behaviour* 205, 68–73.

Islam, S., Gupta, B., Taylor, C.J., Chow, J. and Hoffman, G.R. (2014) Equine-associated maxillofacial injuries: retrospective 5-year analysis. *British Journal of Oral and Maxillofacial Surgery* 52(2), 124–127.

Kruger, L., Hohberg, M., Lehmann, W. and Dresing, K. (2018) Assessing the risk for major injuries in equestrian sports. *British Medical Journal Open Sport and Exercise Medicine* 4(1), e000408.

Kwiatkowska-Stenzel, A., Sowinska, J. and Witkowska, D. (2016) The effect of different bedding materials used in stables on horses behavior. *Journal of Equine Veterinary Science* 42, 57–66.

Lampe, J.F. and Andre, J. (2012) Cross-modal recognition of human individuals in domestic horses (*Equus caballus*). *Animal Cognition* 15(4), 623–630.

Lansade, L., Bonneaua, C., Parias, C. and Biaub, S. (2019) Horse's emotional state and rider safety during grooming practices, a field study. *Applied Animal Behavioural Science* 217, 43–47.

Le Simple, C., Reverchon-Billota, L., Galloux, P., Stompa, M., Boichot, L. *et al.* (2020) Free movement: a key welfare improvement in sport horses? *Applied Animal Behavioural Science* [in press].

Luz, M.P.F., Maia, C.M., Pantoja, J.C.F., Neto, M.C. and Filho, J.N.P.P. (2015) Feeding time and agonistic behaviour in horses: Influence of distance, proportion and height of troughs. *Journal of Equine Veterinary Science* 35(10), 843–848.

McGreevy, P.D. (2007) The advent of equitation science. *The Veterinary Journal* 174(3), 492–500.

McGreevy, P.D., Oddie, C., Burton, F.L. and McLean, A.N. (2009) The horse–human dyad: can we align horse training and handling activities with the equid social ethogram? *The Veterinary Journal* 181(1), 12–18.

McLean, A.N. and McGreevy, P.D. (2010) Horse-training techniques that may defy the principles of learning theory and compromise welfare. *Journal of Veterinary Behavior* 5(4), 187–195.

Millares-Ramirez, E.M. and Le Jeune, S.S. (2019) Girthiness: retrospective study of 37 horses (2004–2016). *Journal of Equine Veterinary Science* 79, 100–104.

Mills, D.S. (1998) Applying learning theory to the management of the horse: the difference between getting it right and getting it wrong. *Equine Veterinary Journal (Supplement)* 27, 44–48.

Paul, S.C. and Stevens, M. (2020) Horse vision and obstacle visibility in horseracing. *Applied Animal Behaviour Science* 222, e104882.

Peters, S.M., Bleijenberg, E.H., van Dierendonck, M.C., van der Harst, J.E. and Spruijt, B.M. (2012) Characterization of anticipatory behaviour in domesticated horses (*Equus caballus*). *Applied Animal Behavioural Science* 138(1-2), 60–69.

Reid, K., Rogers, C.W., Gronqvist, G., Gee, E.K. and Bolwell, C.F. (2017) Anxiety and pain in horses measured by heart rate variability and behavior. *Journal of Veterinary Behavior* 22, 1–6.

Rochais, C., Henry, S. and Hausberger, M. (2018). 'Hay-bags' and 'slow-feeders': testing their impact on horse behaviour and welfare. *Applied Animal Behavioural Science* 198, 52–59.

Rorvang, M.V., Christensen, J.W., Ladewig, J. and McLean, A. (2018) Social learning in horses – fact or fiction? *Frontiers in Veterinary Science* 6(5), 212.

van Balen, P.-J., Barten, D.G., Janssen, L., Fiddelers, A.A.A., Brink, P.R. and Janzing, H.M.J. (2019) Beware of the force of the horse: mechanisms and severity of equestrian-related injuries. *European Journal of Emergency Medicine* 26(2), 133–138.

Verrill, S. and McDonnell, S. (2008) Equal outcomes with and without human-to-horse eye contact when catching horses and ponies in an open pasture. *Journal of Equine Veterinary Science* 28(5), 309–312.

Young, T., Creighton, E., Smith, T. and Hosie, C. (2012) A novel scale of behavioural indicators of stress for use with domestic horses. *Applied Animal Behavioural Science* 140(1-2), 33–43.

Zupan, M., Stuhec, I. and Jordan, D. (2019) The effect of an irregular feeding schedule on equine behavior. *Journal of Applied Animal Welfare Science* 1–8.

3 Groundwork and Foundation Training

Use of the 'Round-pen' Technique

The round-pen phenomenon has been advocated by many diverse trainers and horsepersons over the past few decades, and its use in varying circumstances has been promoted in training programmes, horse shows and demonstrations. It has become a very popular and well-used method in all aspects of a horse's life. However, round-pen does have its distractors and certainly critics. As opinion varies so much with round-pen, this section will explain the current situation through scientific evidence for the reader to express their own judgement of its efficacy.

Round-pen research was introduced to equine literature just over a decade ago working on the suggestion that the act of 'chasing' the horse in the pen until it follows the trainer demonstrated that learning was possibly taking place (Krueger, 2007). When this was tested in an open area after horses had gone through the round-pen training procedure it could not be repeated, therefore it was surmised that horses were not learning to follow the trainer after all. In addition, further research studied the suggestion from round-pen trainers that the way horses respond in the pen is similar to the mare–foal relationship (Warren-Smith and McGreevy, 2008). However, when six mares and their youngstock were watched in a round-pen they only demonstrated chasing behaviour for 0.73% of their time together (Fig. 3.1). There seems to be no evidence to suggest that there is any connection with dominance or the mare–foal relationship, putting into question these two reasons for carrying out round-pen training.

Training outcomes were again investigated 5 years ago, where it was proposed that the learning taking place was not actually from an ethological perspective of natural behaviours but rather based on conditioning and habituation (Henshall and McGreevy, 2014). This would appear to contradict the links with natural horsemanship that purportedly try to mimic horses' natural behaviour to training methods. This idea was further investigated recently when non-expert observers were asked to note behaviours as seen when using natural horsemanship in the round-pen (Wilk and Janczarek, 2015). Interestingly, stress behaviours noted in the round-pen by the observers were not correct, suggesting that observation was difficult. This research also indicated that the first 10 minutes of any session were the most stressful, therefore trainers should be very aware of any intense emotional reactions in this time period (Fig. 3.2).

Researchers studied the aetiology of chasing again recently, examining the differences of frequency of conflict behaviours in horses in round-pen training with professionals and amateurs (Kydd et al., 2017). The amount of chasing by the handlers did not correlate with the horses wanting to follow them, whether they were the experienced trainers or not. However, even though fewer conflict behaviours were observed with professionals, it was recommended that those involved at any level with round-pen training must make sure they have sufficient knowledge to recognize how to use negative reinforcement to try to reduce the incidence of such adverse behaviour. Education of learning theory also came into focus with the most recent paper to date on round-pen, where safety issues for horse and handler were raised if trainers did not understand their actions by way of learning theory or inadequately applied this understanding (Fenner et al., 2019). It was reported that conflict behaviours were evidenced, indicating that those horses demonstrating those behaviours were highly aroused and as such putting themselves and their handlers into danger. The other issue discussed related round-pen to lungeing, where chasing behaviour is also evidenced in some cases and could lead to detrimental learning in horses where punishment is used inadvertently by handlers who do not understand learning theory adequately.

The research so far appears to point towards possible problems with the round-pen method,

© R. Scofield 2020. *Solving Equine Behaviour Problems* (R. Scofield)

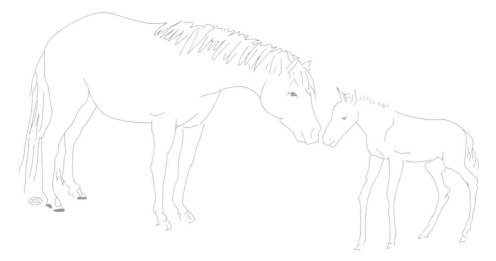

Fig. 3.1. When mares and foals are released into a round-pen there is very limited observation of the mare chasing the foal.

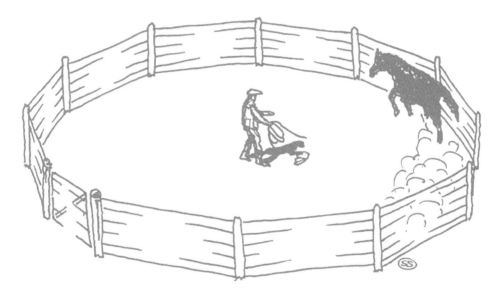

Fig. 3.2. Round-pen training seems to be coaching the horse to follow the handler; however, the confusion with the use of negative reinforcement and punishment appears all too apparent when it is studied closely.

particularly if handlers and trainers do not really understand or are uninformed about the use of learning theory in training. It is wise at present to advise handlers and trainers to limit their use of the technique, unless they are fully conversant with how learning theory plays its part in the chasing and following of horses seen in the method. Without knowledge, and the application of this through experience, it does appear that many horses may suffer adverse effects from having this technique included in their foundation training, daily life or indeed retraining.

A Note on Training Aids

The popularity of training aids – those artificial devices that have been invented to help handlers and owners control their horses – has possibly never been greater. There is some evidence to suggest these devices are utilized by a majority of leisure horse owners (78%) to help them deal with problem behaviours (Hockenhull and Creighton, 2012). There are also reports of the use of training aids contributing to likelihood of discomfort and increasing the frequency of conflict behaviour, both of which should be avoided if possible by owners and trainers. However, certain items such as the Pessoa®, Dually® pressure headcollar (Fig. 3.3) and draw reins are often used by professionals too. This section will look at some of the most popular to be investigated by researchers in equitation science to enable choices to be made, or at least caution advised.

Draw reins and martingales work on the same principle of holding the horse's head in a downward position rotated from the poll distally, but draw reins, due to their construction, have the ability to allow a handler or rider to apply a far greater amount of pressure (Fig. 3.4). Due to this they have also been linked to the origin of pain in some horses (Rhodin *et al.*, 2005). Draw reins act directly on the bit, so the rider can use pressure to force the head and neck into the desirable position of the 2nd/3rd vertebrae as the highest point, with the aspect of the nasal plane caudally positioned and characterized as 'behind the vertical' (Toft *et al.*, 2020). Interestingly, when comparing

dressage horses in 1994 with those in 2008, a significant increase in horses in 2008 were seen with head positions behind the vertical (Lashley *et al.*, 2014). Even though the Fédération Equestre International (FEI), the body governing most horse sports in the world except horse-racing, advocates that the head position should be somewhat in advance of the vertical, this has apparently not been promoted in dressage scoring (FEI, 2020). It is still favourable for riders and trainers to crave the 'behind the vertical' head position, although there is a whole other debate on the detrimental effects of using hyperflexion, or as it is known 'rollkur', to gain this desirable image.

Intriguingly, the 'behind the vertical' head position seems to influence the position of the forelegs rather than the hind (Weishaupt *et al.*, 2006) (Fig. 3.5), where moving parallel to the forelegs is supposedly desired in dressage tests (commonly termed 'tracking-up') (Fig. 3.6). If the horse is forced into this position with training aids such as draw reins, it appears to lack the uphill motion and collection afforded by those horses trained without artificial aids. There is also concern about the

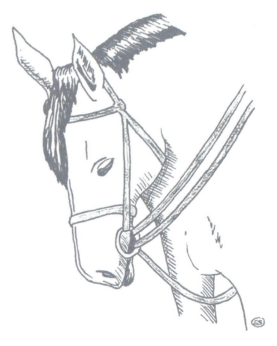

Fig. 3.4. Draw reins in use while a horse is being ridden – the rider holds both sets of reins and should be experienced enough to be able to use them independently only when needed.

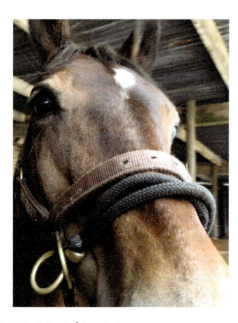

Fig. 3.3. A Dually® headcollar.

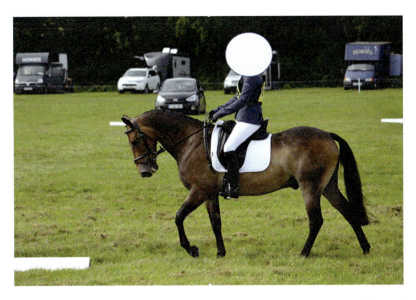

Fig. 3.5. A horse in the 'behind-the-vertical' head position – it can be clearly seen that the poll is not the highest point and the nasal plane does not follow a vertical line.

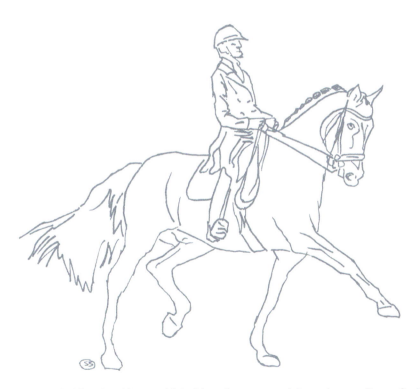

Fig. 3.6. A behind-the-vertical head position established from the overuse of draw reins or a Pessoa® with no release of pressure may also develop a lack of parallel movement between the front and hind legs.

possible implications of welfare issues, as many studies report a rise in conflict behaviours, heart rate and other indicators (McGreevy, 2007; von Borstel *et al.*, 2009). However, the incidence of using these methods including draw reins and hyperflexion are so popular and appear to save time in the preparation of young stock that they are employed on a regular basis. Concern possibly occurs when those trainers applying such artificial aids use them improperly, and also perhaps without understanding negative reinforcement. In addition to this, in the case of the Pessoa©, they have grown in popularity for a greater number of horse owners who may very well be without the correct training and are influenced by trends to try them out on their own horses (Hockenhull and Creighton, 2012).

The Pessoa® lungeing system has been studied to a limited extent in the field of equitation science, although as with other methods there is a need for further experiments to take place. The Pessoa® is quite a complicated system of ropes and pulleys, designed to act on the horse's bit in a downward direction with pressure originating from the hind legs. The device can be altered to become more, or less, severe and is valued anecdotally across complementary therapy in its use for strengthening the back and manipulating the vertebrae. In research, it has been reported that the Pessoa® does act to shorten the stride of the horse, therefore possibly promoting a rounding of the horse's back (Walker *et al.*, 2013). However, it is also known to reduce activity in muscles associated with back function, perhaps due to this shortened stride (Tabor and Williams, 2018), so it is uncertain how much of a favourable influence the use of this device has as a therapy tool.

Another aspect of the Pessoa® is the action on the bit, where, as previously mentioned, the pressure is relayed through a system of ropes and pulleys. It has been stated that this pressure acts on the bars of the mouth via the bit on each stride, potentially nullifying any feature of the device to utilize negative reinforcement correctly (McLean and McGreevy, 2010). If there is continuous and irregular pressure with no reduction correlating to response and reward, there is the real danger of psychological problems developing for the horse involved. Due to this possibility, it was recommended by Walker *et al.* (2013) that the device should be fitted with this in mind; however, the irregular pressure on each stride would not alter by fitting the Pessoa® any differently.

Headcollar types and designs have received hardly any attention in research, but since the advent of studies looking at nosebands it is possible this may change in the future. The one headcollar where some research was carried out is the Dually®, where the noseband of the headcollar has two separate attachments: one has no movement and the other can be tightened to employ pressure to the facial structures (Fig. 3.7). It was designed to help handlers control horses by putting more pressure on these sensitive structures than a normal headcollar, enabling the handler to exert more force on the animal than is possible using a fixed-strap headcollar alone. This can make horses more amenable to what the handler requires, as less pressure is used to instruct the horse on what the handler wants. As this action is escalating the ability to cause pain to the horse, the experiment was designed to measure levels of discomfort between using the Dually® pressure strap and the fixed strap as a control (Ijichi *et al.*, 2018). Findings suggested that there was an increase in pain indicators in horses where the pressure strap was used, but controversially these horses were also judged not to have displayed more amenable behaviour than those using only the fixed strap.

Evidently more research is needed, not only with the Dually®, due to its popularity (Fig. 3.8), but also other types of headcollar such as those with very thin rope straps known anecdotally as 'humane headcollars'. It is possible that there is nothing humane about them, since physics appears to suggest a thinner strap must exert more pressure, not less. Also, there appear to be headcollar designs that incorporate metal fixings on pressure points, perhaps even more so demonstrating the erroneousness of the anecdotal name. It is therefore suggested that horses in foundation training, retraining or any other education should be undergoing a programme of correct leading, with a plain headcollar, progressing to groundwork using learning theory as a basis for these programmes.

Problems Investigated

Introduction to novel objects

A part of any horse's training involves the introduction of novel, or new, objects. These could range from everyday objects that the horse has probably encountered all its life, such as headcollars, buckets, grooming kits, to unusual items like cars and other traffic, and perhaps different farm animals. Possibly

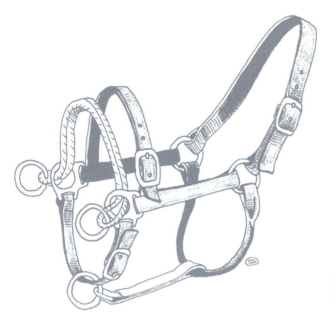

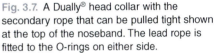
Fig. 3.7. A Dually® head collar with the secondary rope that can be pulled tight shown at the top of the noseband. The lead rope is fitted to the O-rings on either side.

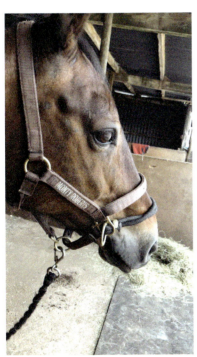
Fig. 3.8. Example of a Dually® head collar.

the best environment for a foal to grow up in is one where it is carefully exposed to many objects, so a long period of habituation occurs and continues throughout its life (Fig. 3.9). Companionship of other herd members is vital at these times, particularly if there is a mixture of ages and experiences for the foal to relate to. Early walking out with other horses is useful to introduce the youngster to the many different forms of traffic it may encounter in the future, and, as discussed, a horse's ability to use generalization in its learning perfectly adapts it for this to be exploited in training.

With an older horse exposure to novel objects can occur at any time, and for the owner the appearance of something the horse has not encountered before – if completely different to anything else they have seen – can be problematic. Studies on horses' reactions to novel objects using various training methods appear to work well with less stress (Marsboll and Christensen, 2015; Christensen, 2016). Horses exposed to novel objects on a voluntary basis rather than using a negative reinforcer like pressure-release are less stressed and habituate to the objects more quickly (Christensen, 2013). This research would appear to suggest that, to reduce fear, either a voluntary approach or a positively reinforced method should be used. If a rider suddenly discovers a novel object while out hacking, the best method would indeed be to let the horse approach the object in its own time, and under a voluntary basis. The use of coercive tactics such as employing a whip or kicking as punishment will incur all the adverse connotations that this form of training brings. Negative reinforcement

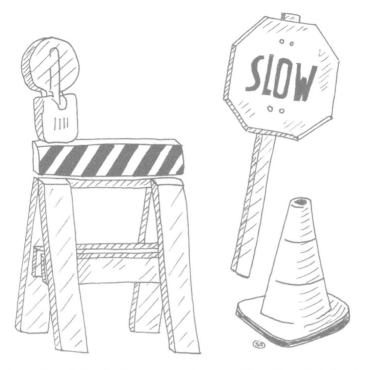

Fig. 3.9. Novel objects experienced when hacking can comprise many different items, including those used in roadworks.

can be employed but this will raise stress levels, so may not be the correct method to use if the horse is already stressed through the novel situation.

These ridden occurrences can also be dangerous, with the possibility of the horse bolting, or at least shying or spinning round – both of which behaviours are dealt with later. However, if a novel object is experienced when the horse is being led, the same methods apply, and voluntary exploration appears to be the most prudent solution (Fig. 3.10). Indeed, with young horses, or horses that are in the process of being retrained to better accept novel objects and scary situations, a training programme can be put in place utilizing this method. Access to a school or arena makes for a safer environment, where the horse can be led in-hand to various objects on a regular basis in its retraining programme. Other novel objects are more problematic, such as traffic, and especially tractors, which are a well-known fearful object amongst horse-riders. These may be better dealt with using classical conditioning alongside the voluntary approach, and this method is explained in the case studies. The use of positive reinforcement is also discussed in another pertinent case study included in this section.

Key points

- Research suggests that a voluntary approach using either positive reinforcement or classical conditioning reduces stress and habituates horses faster.
- Using punishment, for instance a whip or kicking to force the animal past a novel object, appears to raise stress levels and could be dangerous in a horse already about to bolt or spin around.
- It is a good idea to expose young horses to novel objects such as traffic in their foundation training.
- Negative reinforcement can also be employed, but probably better not used if the horse is displaying signs of stress.

Take-home message

In a horse already stressed and indicating it may bolt or spin, punishment in the form of whips and kicking is clearly not the answer.

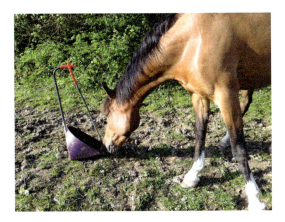

Fig. 3.10. Horses will explore anything they consider a novel object, even if they have been introduced to them before.

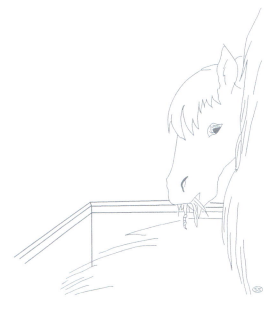

Fig. 3.11. The horse readily ate from the tractor trailer, owing to its strong motivation with its food.

Case study 1

The first case study illustrates how sometimes solving behavioural problems is all about using everyday situations to provide feasible training opportunities. A gelding of around 9 years old had just been purchased and it was known by the new owner that he was fearful of tractors. Buying this horse was a risk, but with retraining the problem was surmountable at the particular livery yard where the animal was going to be kept. This was because the horses were fed hay off the farmer's tractor trailer, and he had a set route he followed every morning to deliver it into the fields. The horses with less fear approached the trailer and stole hay from the back – while the farmer was tipping the trailer! When the gelding was introduced to the field the owner watched carefully the next morning to see what happened. As expected, the new horse was extremely fearful and cantered off when it saw the vehicle. Over the next few days the owner watched as the horse became more motivated to get to the hay first and overcome its fear through classical conditioning. By the end of the week the horse was pushing in to get its share of the hay and seemed to be over its fear (Fig. 3.11).

The next stage was to test this in the yard, to see if the horse would generalize the tractor within different environments. It worked perfectly – the horse was rather excited to see the tractor, and when another differently coloured tractor was driven in there was no reaction other than great interest. Ridden work was next, and again the

retraining appeared to have solved the problem. This was extended to hacking out and having the odd tractor or large, noisy lorry passing the pair. This technique using classical conditioning to encourage less fearful responses has appeared to work particularly well on several occasions.

Case study 2

The second case study involving novel objects concerned an endurance pony that was terrified of quad bikes (small four-wheeled motorcycles). In this case the behaviourist remembered a very similar situation and decided to employ the same tactic. A quad bike from a farm local to the pony was engaged and the driver was given a bag of horse treat of the type favoured by the pony. As the animal was particularly fearful of this vehicle, and these are encountered all the time in the endurance discipline (ridden by marshals), it was decided to replicate this situation as much as possible. The pony was ridden by the rider with two other herd members in a safe field, and the quad bike was asked to approach very slowly and stop before getting too close. One of the horses was ridden up to the quad and the driver gave him a treat. This happened with the other horse too, and then the quad drove away. The riders went a little further down the track and repeated the process. On the fourth time the pony wanted to approach the quad, therefore using the voluntary approach, and finally took a treat from the driver. The exercise was repeated a few times a week, until the sight of a quad bike was rather appetitive to the animal, and the first endurance ride after the retraining was a total success. The only downfall to this method was that the pony did really want to approach any quad bike it saw; however, over time, once the treat-based approach was stopped the reaction to the stimulus would naturally become extinct.

Clipping

The action of clipping a horse is carried out for many reasons and is usually a normal part of a young horse's foundation training (Fig. 3.12). Fear of clipping in an older horse is generally a reaction to something aversive happening in a clipping session, but the same methods can be used in foundation training as would be employed here. Indeed, a fear reaction to clipping can be based on many factors of the clipping process, such as heat, vibration, noise, the electric cable in some models and also snagging the skin if the horse is still wet or muddy or oil is not used properly on the blades. Any, or a combination, of these elements may cause problem behaviour if the horse associates pain or discomfort with the action of clipping. Another point to make concerns the use of sedatives to clip horses: unfortunately these can cause horses to sweat, thus making the clipping process even more different, so it is advised that the horse should be retrained rather than medicated.

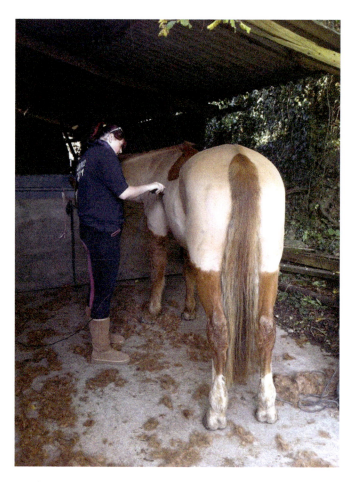

Fig. 3.12. It often appears advantageous to clip the offside or right side of a horse first, leaving the nearside, or left side, to which they are more accustomed, for the final adjustments.

There are a few different approaches to desensitize a horse so that it will accept clippers again, and each can start with a different trigger. If it is possible to ascertain which element the horse is most afraid of, this can be tackled first. For example, if the noise is what appears to make the horse fearful, a recording of the sound may prove useful, or a horse being clipped in the same yard on a regular basis near the fearful horse may help. By desensitizing the horse to the sound of the clippers it begins to lose its fear, but this needs to be completed in successive approximations (shaping), with a cool-off period if the horse becomes too stressed. However, it is usually very difficult to determine what the trigger is, so retraining would normally consist of a holistic approach to all the factors clipping might entail. A curious note to mention here includes anecdotal evidence for clipping to begin on the right-hand side of the horse – what might be described as the side horses are least touched (leading, mounting for example). If the horse is going to get frustrated at standing for so long, or is going to react, the 'hardest' side is already done, and the 'easier' left-hand side is left to complete. Before this advice can be given, research needs to be carried out.

The first part of the retraining would include establishing how afraid the horse is, and then tailoring the programme to take this into account. The severity of the problem will affect the treatment, so some horses may need preliminary training with small hand-held clippers, which are quieter and operate with no cable, to eliminate some of the issues (Fig. 3.13). The horse may need initial sessions just being rubbed with the clippers turned off, gradually progressing to turning them on. The horse can then be adjusted to having small areas clipped and progressing to the large clippers over a period of time, eventually leading to a horse that can be clipped with no fear. Nevertheless, some horses require much more time, with other learning theories incorporated into their retraining. An example of this would be using overshadowing, where, as discussed in Chapter 1, the horse is trained to lead correctly with negative reinforcement, and then is asked to move forwards and backwards while the clippers are placed on its body. This method does work surprisingly well; the forwards and backwards movement is lessened as the horse loses its aversive behavioural reaction to the clipper stimulus.

Key points

- Systematic desensitization is a must when retraining a horse to accept clipping (Fig. 3.14).
- It is best to use a combination of methods to overcome the fear as it may exist for many different reasons.
- Using a holistic approach seems to work best when dealing with clipper issues.

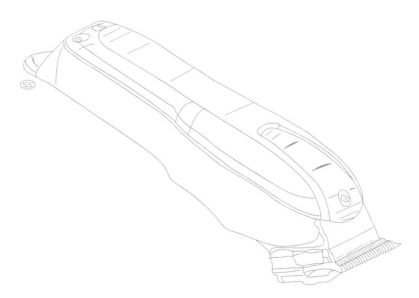

Fig. 3.13. Small hand-held clippers may prove useful in retraining.

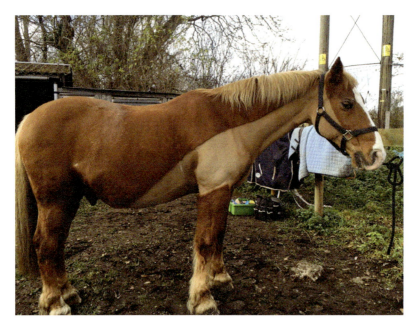

Fig. 3.14. An older pony with a low trace clip avoiding its sensitive hindquarter area and observing the amount of stress the horse can cope with, even if trained with desensitization.

Take-home message

Using a combination of theories seems to provide the best solutions, so overshadowing and shaping within the umbrella of systematic desensitization is recommended.

Case study

A very hypersensitive cob was proving rather difficult to clip at a riding school and had become worse, until it could not be approached at all by someone with clippers. This was obviously a severe reaction to clipping, but unusual as it had developed over a period of time. The horse was quite reactive to handling on the ground, and when ridden, but could jump exceptionally well so was kept on at the school. The first advice was to begin to retrain correct leading, in case this was needed as part of overshadowing. However, over a period of instruction to stable staff and some observations, it was soon very apparent that a quick solution was not going to work for this particular horse. Therefore, a programme was set in place with a strict protocol for every person handling the horse to follow, including correct leading, calm schooling and hacking and to take time over grooming rather

than the rushed sessions that usually happened. The reduction in stressful situations for the horse in its daily life began to have effect, and then the clipping training began. The horse showed a fear reaction to a horse being clipped in the next stable, so this was done at the end of the five-horse block on a regular basis. Staff always carried a vibrating toothbrush in their pocket when handling the horse (Fig. 3.15) – not to use it but for the vibration and noise to become a regular happening.

Over a period of a month the horse went through this holistic treatment, and at the end of the period it was visited again and battery clippers were carried into the stable. The lack of reaction to them was very pleasing and the horse proceeded to let them be used just below his withers. From then on, the programme consisted of staff using the battery clippers and gradually progressing to clipping the horse with a trace clip (Fig. 3.16), which is one of the least invasive clips. The horse never advanced to having its face or its groin area clipped again, but the trace was enough to enable the horse to return to work appropriately in the school. Indeed, the whole process had seemed to calm the horse considerably, so it did not spook as readily on hacks, nor did it rush over jumps as much as previously. A holistic approach such as used on this horse appeared to affect its whole life, not just the issue with the clippers. More research is needed concerning the aspects of this case.

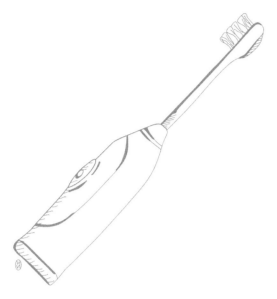

Fig. 3.15. A vibrating toothbrush will imitate the sound and feel of clippers but in a far less aversive manner than even small clippers.

Rugging

As with clipping, rugging should be part of every young horse's foundation training, but problems can develop in the older horse if an accident happens in the field or stable. A combination of systematic desensitization, perhaps used with positive reinforcement, usually provides the best solution for rugging problems, again with the speed of the retraining being determined by managing the stress levels of the horse carefully. Using a bath towel or a small blanket as a 'starter' rug is useful in retraining, as is exploiting a motivational reward system when the horse stands still once the towel is placed over its withers (Fig. 3.17). As horses can develop 'rug phobias', but be perfectly able to tolerate a saddlecloth, the substitute starter rug can be placed on the withers first. It could be folded, and then unfolded to make it bigger and cover a larger area of the body over a period of time dictated by the reactions of the horse.

Rug straps can also be the cause of problems (Fig. 3.18), and again the same method of making the whole process appetitive with reward-based desensitization may be employed. Reward does not necessarily have to entail treats but can be vocal or by scratching the horse's favourite place. Hind-leg

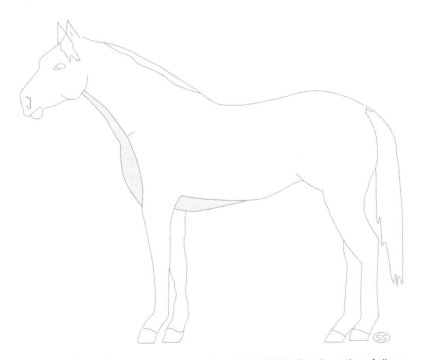

Fig. 3.16. A very low trace clip could be used on a horse when desensitizing it to the action of clippers.

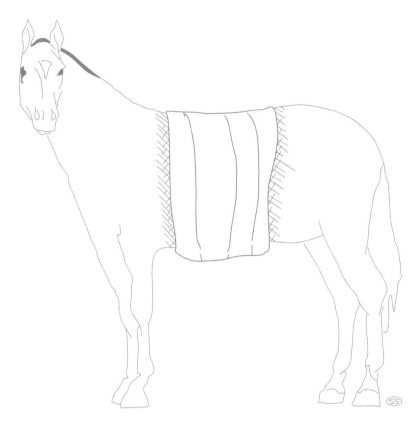

Fig. 3.17. For a very fearful horse a towel could be used as a small substitute rug while in the process of desensitization.

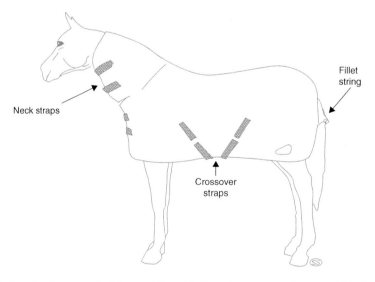

Fig. 3.18. An illustration showing a rug that does not have hind-leg straps – sometimes useful for horses that are sensitive in this area.

straps can be particularly problematic, but there are types of rugs that do not have these, so they may be a solution. It is important to make sure that the rug is a good fit and that all the straps are secure, particularly in the case of a horse being retrained, so that no further issues develop.

Key points

- Make sure any retraining is started with a smaller and easier-to-manage bath towel or blanket.
- Using reward-based desensitization appears to have very beneficial effects.

Take-home message

In order to avoid complications developing, it is advisable to have rugs that fit correctly (Fig. 3.19) and that do not have broken straps.

Case study

A mature gelding was the subject of this case study, and the problem had emerged after the owner used

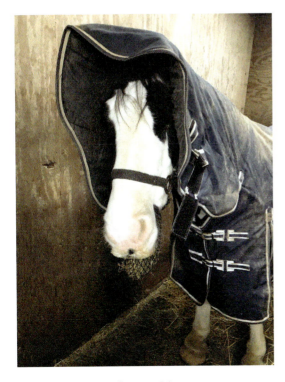

Fig. 3.19. Rugs must fit correctly!

a hood on the horse in the field to protect it from mud. It was the type with eye holes, and unfortunately had got snagged on something and was pulled over one of the horse's eyes so it could not see properly. When the horse was brought in, it was quickly realized that any type of rug over its body had become a real issue, as the animal seemed to have learnt this was the same as the hood.

The process of desensitization began, and this time started with a blanket over the rump of the horse as the only place it would tolerate it – possibly due to the issue developing on the head at first. General protocol was followed, and the horse in this case was given its normal feed and fed from its usual bucket at the same time as the blanket retraining took place. This procedure was suggested as another way to calm the horse and reduce stress levels and the decision to use the method in this circumstance worked very well. Over a week, the sessions were carried out at feeding time and the horse was rugged up by the end of the period with little stress or complication. This was a situation where the training needed to happen as quickly as possible, because of weather conditions and the horse being unable to be turned out due to the lack of a rug. Solving this particular case involved as usual some thinking and consideration – rarely is there a situation with behaviour problems where there is not.

Tacking-up

Bridle and bit

As part of foundation training the bridle should follow the headcollar, where the horse has had a period of desensitization to place the headcollar on correctly, possibly motivated by reward. In cases where feral horses or those that have never been properly handled need to be trained, methods of reward usually involve extensive sessions with feed buckets and headcollars. Once a horse has accepted a headcollar, the bridle leather itself should not pose a problem: it is the bit that needs prudent introduction (Fig. 3.20). For a horse that has a problem with tacking up and specifically a bridle, the origin might be in the mouth (where someone has inadvertently or on purpose tugged on the reins and jabbed the mouth) or possibly with the headpiece. The expression 'head-shy' is often used to describe an animal that has had aversive application of force on its head, or ears, or has been in an accident. As the head is reached for to slide the bridle into place, the horse backs away or throws its head up in remembered pain.

Head-shy horses can successfully be retrained using positive reinforcement with desensitization, where each stage is rewarded and if the horse becomes stressed the process is taken back a stage. It is important to make the whole process appetitive to the individual horse, especially the insertion of the bit if one is used. If the problem was caused by mouth damage, there is scope with a head-shy horse to use a bitless bridle; however, in strong hands they are not necessarily any better than a bridle with a bit and can contribute to conflict behaviours (Kienapfel *et al.*, 2014). For those that have problems with the headpiece and the ears in particular, a useful part of the retraining protocol might be to start by scratching or touching the ears before the bridle is put anywhere near the horse. It is a matter

of dissecting what stimulus triggers the reaction, and then working to eliminate the fearful responses of the horse by introducing positive reinforcement at every stage. As the bridle is probably the most important communication tool for the rider, it should be used for this purpose and not as any form of punishment. When leading with the bridle it is critical not to be tempted to jerk on the reins and use it as a tool for punishment. Indeed, when riding, the signals given with the reins should also be executed with care and this will be discussed later.

Call-outs for bitting are not uncommon, and generally involve the owner or rider having to progress to stronger bits due to their horse becoming unresponsive, possibly when undertaking more exciting disciplines such as hunting or cross-country. Certainly, many riders keep a stronger bit for these activities, and this works perfectly well, so the case study below is not necessarily for them, but for the rider who has found that the progression of using stronger bits has not worked. It is common for these riders to trial a bit that is believed to cause a higher poll pressure, in order to try to bring back control of the head to the rider; however, even simple snaffles have a moderate action on the poll (Cross *et al.*, 2017) (Fig. 3.21). It is important at this point to understand that a rider who pulls incessantly on any bit (or bitless bridle) can cause trauma to the horse's mouth, whereas a light-handed rider can use the most severe bit with no distress experienced by the horse.

Stronger bits can be described as a regression from using a more comfortable bit for the horse, such as a snaffle, which is reported to cause fewer lesions to the bars of the mouth than a curb-style bit (Bjornsdottir *et al.*, 2014). When it is brought into action the straighter shape of the snaffle bit causes less pressure on the bars of the mouth and also the poll, ensuring a lesser chance of abrasions or injury (Fig. 3.22). Anecdotally, riders have used snaffles as a starter bit in foundation training, only using stronger bits such as curbs or those with a

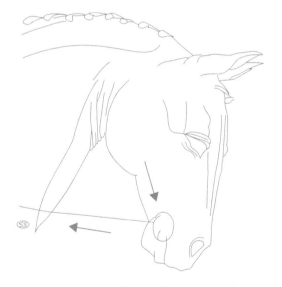

Fig. 3.20. A simple snaffle bit still exerts a certain amount of pressure on the poll of the horse.

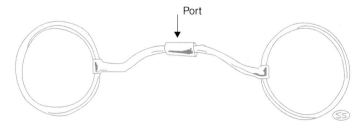

Port

Fig. 3.21. A loose-ring snaffle with a moveable convex port, giving extra room for the tongue.

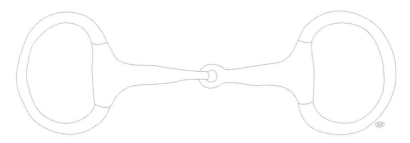

Fig. 3.22. An eggbutt (fixed) snaffle bit with jointed mouthpiece.

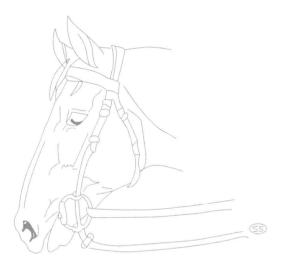

Fig. 3.23. A gag bit – a rope is threaded through the bit ring and attached to a secondary rein to provide access to extra poll pressure for the rider.

'port' (a curve in the metal that extends cranially) when the horse appears to start to ignore the original snaffle bit. Experience of behavioural cases now seems to suggest that actually reducing the perceived strength of a bit and retraining the horse to properly understand what signals it is receiving is far more successful than regressing to stronger bits and types of noseband (Fig. 3.23).

BITLESS BRIDLES. Bitless bridles have perhaps been in existence since horses were domesticated, with evidence of bits seen in many places across the world. Many types of bitless bridle exist, and in many cultures, with the UK predominantly using a type known as the Hackamore, which acts on the nasal bone instead of the bars of the mouth as a bit does. Since the advent of the idea of natural horsemanship, bits have been

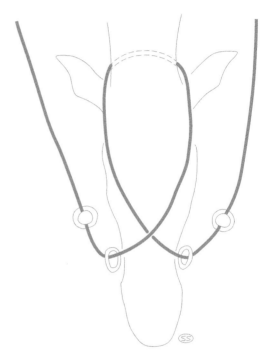

Fig. 3.24. The Dr Cook® cross-under bitless bridle demonstrating the action of the reins to squeeze the whole head as an aid to stopping and turning.

somewhat vilified, and suggestions have been made to replace them with various new bitless bridles. One of these has been the subject of contradictory research (Cook and Mills, 2009; Scofield and Randle, 2012, 2013) working on a system of cross-under straps to put pressure on the whole head (Fig. 3.24). There has been anecdotal comment about how quick-releasing this system is, and whether the correct application of negative reinforcement is unable to give the vital pressure-release, therefore turning the pressure into punishment (Fig. 3.25). One of the case studies below looks at a possibility of this happening.

Often replacing a bitted bridle with a bitless one can (anecdotally) be enough to solve bit-related behavioural problems, but it is pertinent to note that it should not be used as a solution for every single mouthing issue, as pressure on the nasal bones is still pressure and has the potential to cause injury if used incorrectly. In research it has been reported that there was no difference in lesions around horses' lips regardless of whether they were wearing a bitted or bitless bridle (Uldahl and Clayton, 2019). Certainly, as mentioned, using a bitless bridle that works on the premise of pressure on the nasal bones that is released very quickly due to lack of any tightening device may indeed prove to be the solution for horses that do not readily accept bits in their mouths. One example of this is the bosal (Fig. 3.26), where a pre-formed piece of leather is shaped around the nasal bone and the reins join it under the chin. When pressure is exerted on the reins, and then released, there is no tightening of straps and so pressure is released immediately.

With bitted bridles, advice is often given to increase the strength of a bit in a horse that is beginning to ignore signals from the rider. However, increasing pressure in this way acts only to further deaden the response from the horse, indicating that a return to a lighter bit under controlled conditions may be better (see case studies below). To date, equine ruling bodies are still very reluctant to raise the ban on bitless bridles being used in certain disciplines like dressage, due to the conflicting reports, and more research is needed to pinpoint where the problems, if any exist, are occurring.

NOSEBANDS. There are many different types of noseband, the simplest being a plain strap that fits around the nose and is known as a cavesson. This noseband can be tightened, but as it is quite high up on the horse's facial structure it will not itself have very much action on the mouth. A very common type of cavesson, fitted lower down towards the muzzle, is called the 'crank', which acts on a system of pulleys to enable it to be very tightly applied. The crank quickly gained popularity, and in the Netherlands it is reported as being used by 82% of dressage riders, though by only 6% of showjumpers (Visser *et al.*, 2019) (Fig. 3.27). Perhaps the ability to tighten the noseband has led to its adoption, as in the same study 45.7% riders reported that their choice of noseband was due to its ease of use. The 'flash' noseband, which consists of an extra strap joined

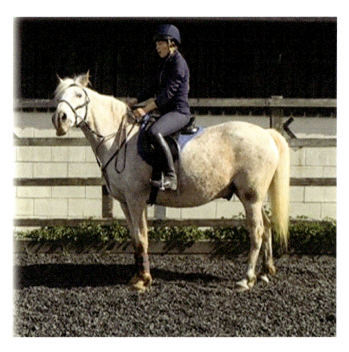

Fig. 3.25. Experimentation found that conflict behaviours were displayed in halt tests whilst horses wore the bitless bridle.

to the cavesson and then being strapped below the bit to act in the same way as a crank, i.e. to keep the mouth closed, is also a popular choice but it exerts a significantly increased amount of pressure

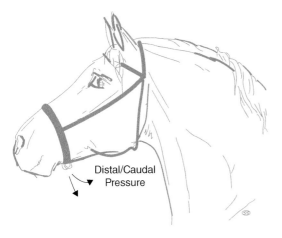

Fig. 3.26. A bosal bitless bridle illustrating the downward and backward pressure on the horse's nasal plane, but having the ability to release immediately, due to the lack of any tightening straps.

when measured against a plain cavesson (Murray *et al.*, 2015).

The noseband is suggested to try to eliminate oral movement in dressage horses, as this is marked down in dressage tests across the world. However, if the horse's natural instinct is to chew to remove foreign bodies in the oral cavity (Doherty *et al.*, 2017b), then perhaps the bit itself should be examined for any issues it is causing. The action of the tongue also dispels pressure in the mouth (Manfredi *et al.*, 2009), adding to the necessity for this movement and providing evidence for bit pressure issues. Also, the motion of chewing and licking is correlated with response to, and is a sign of, a stressful event (Henshall and McGreevy, 2014; Doherty *et al.*, 2017a), so actually stopping this instinct with a tight noseband is possibly detrimental to the health of the animal. Perhaps due to these welfare concerns, investigation into the use of nosebands has arisen in many contemporary research studies. There appears to be evidence of real physical issues when restrictive nosebands are used on horses, concerning cheek ulceration and possible bone deformation (Crago *et al.*, 2019; Uldahl and Clayton, 2019). Studies examining the tightness of

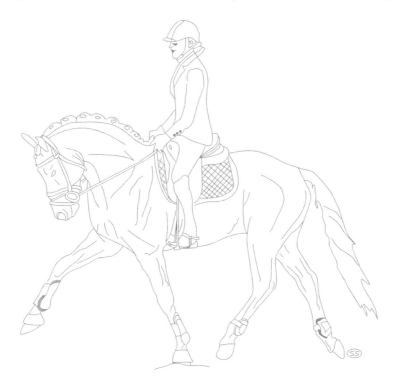

Fig. 3.27. Tight nosebands are more often seen on dressage horses.

nosebands have been conducted with measures of eye temperature rising when nosebands were tighter (McGreevy *et al.*, 2012; Fenner *et al.*, 2016), heart rate rising (Fenner *et al.* 2016) and skin temperature rising (McGreevy *et al.*, 2012), possibly indicating reduction of blood supply.

Countries in Europe, an example being the Netherlands, have instigated regulations making testing for nosebands that are 'too tight' mandatory in some competitions (Visser *et al.*, 2019). In the Netherlands, 98% of riders were aware of the new regulations brought into force, although only 54.5% agreed with them (Visser *et al.*, 2019). Oddly, 62% then stated that they believed the rules would improve equine welfare. In the UK, there are recommendations, but these contradict the scientific research available and appear to give the wrong instruction about how tightness should be measured. According to studies, the noseband should be measured on the nasal plane, not in a lateral placement as suggested by some equitation organizations, as this merely crushes the tissue into the cheek, preventing a genuine measurement (Fig. 3.28).

Present advice from one of the latest studies appears to suggest that nosebands should be worn, but should be loose enough to allow two fingers to be inserted between the nasal plane and the noseband itself (Doherty *et al.*, 2017b) (Fig. 3.29). This enables the horse to perform natural oral behaviours of chewing but allows for some restriction as suggested to keep the bridle and bit

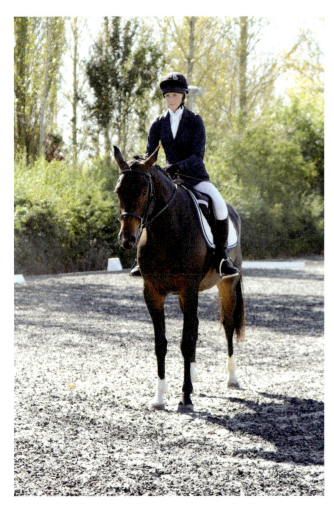

Fig. 3.28. In the future, all dressage horses may need to have their nosebands measured for tightness.

Chapter 3

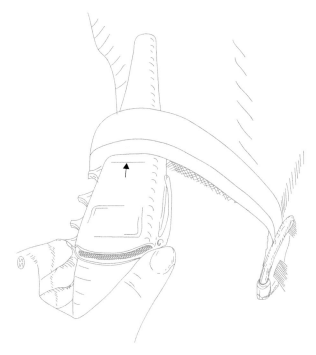

Fig. 3.29. A simple noseband tightness measuring device invented by the International Society for Equitation Science (adapted from www.equitationscience.com).

in a stable position, as riding completely without a noseband also appears to cause ulcers. Regrettably for the welfare of the horse, as stated, any undue movement of the mouth is marked down by dressage judges, so until awarding of points under dressage rules is changed or adapted, riders in countries that have not banned the use of tight nosebands may continue to use them. Until other organizations investigate changing these regulations, it is possible the proven detrimental effects of this part of the bridle will still be causing many problems into the future.

Saddles

As with the bridle, the fitting of the saddle and girth takes place in foundation training. Issues can arise with the girth, where horses have had previous experiences with rubbing caused by an ill-fitted or dirty item or a lack of thorough grooming. The young horse should be introduced slowly to the saddle and girth, using the same methods and gradually desensitizing them. Some training methods do advocate putting the saddle on straight away and tightening the girth, then lungeing the horse using habituation rather than systematic desensitization as advised above. This method works, but it does tend to cause the horse heightened levels of stress through flooding and may instigate bucking and rearing, all of which can cause injury to the horse or the handler and potentially create adverse learning experiences. Therefore, it is suggested that less stressful methods are used, particularly for the horse that develops a problem with the saddle or girth where stress is already an issue. Using the method of systematic desensitization can also involve steps developed from foundation training, where many youngsters are introduced to the experience of wearing a 'roller' before they graduate to a saddle (Fig, 3.30). A roller is a wide strip of leather or fabric tightened around the girth, sometimes with rings and attachment points for other gadgets. It is tightened like a girth and can give the horse further time to adjust to the feel of tension around its belly without the weight of a saddle. These are also very useful in retraining and can be an easy step to the saddle for some fearful subjects.

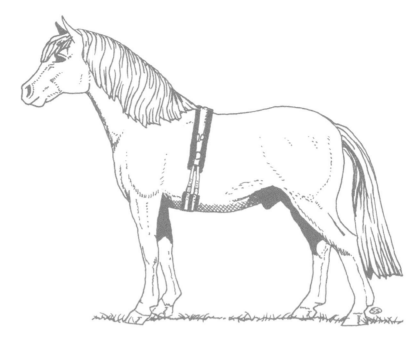

Fig. 3.30. A roller fitted to a pony.

When using methods to reintroduce the saddle, consider that there may be problems involving the stirrups and remember it is important to make sure they are secured properly on the leathers if this is a complication. As training progresses, stirrups can be let down gradually to make contact with the horse's flanks, enabling all the stimuli with the saddle to be experienced. Once the horse is comfortable with the saddle, a rider can be reintroduced, perhaps with handlers present in case there is any reaction. Some people involved in foundation training use dummies on the saddles to simulate a rider, but there is no evidence to indicate that this is better than a balanced and experienced rider. An advantage of using a rider is their ability to mount calmly and carefully, and also be prepared to put weight into the saddle gradually, rather than habituation with the whole burden at once.

THE PHENOMENON OF THE 'COLD-BACKED' HORSE. Other problems can occur with the saddle, including the condition known as 'cold-backed', which manifests as the horse 'sinking' or 'dipping' when the rider lowers themselves into the saddle, or momentary difficulty with movement on mounting (Fig. 3.31). There is no evidence to explain what these signs represent, although there have been suggestions that they are linked to badly fitting saddles or foundation training (De Cocq *et al.*, 2004). Whether it is an issue of remembered pain, temperament or actual discomfort at the time is unknown. If a horse presents with this issue, there is an urgent need for a full veterinary examination to eliminate any present problems. However, in cases where this has been done there might appear to be no existing problem yet the cold-backed horse continues to sink down on mounting. There are devices available on the market aimed to warm up the back before the horse is tacked up, but these lack any empirical evidence and it is still unclear if warmth is an issue, despite the connotations from the name. Once veterinary checks have been made, horses like these can still be ridden, but may benefit from being led around before mounting, and certainly need a sympathetic rider to work out the most practical way to work with the problem.

GASTRIC ULCERS. Another possible medical issue that may well contribute to saddling problems can be the incidence of gastric ulcers causing pain in the girthing area (Fig. 3.32). Research found

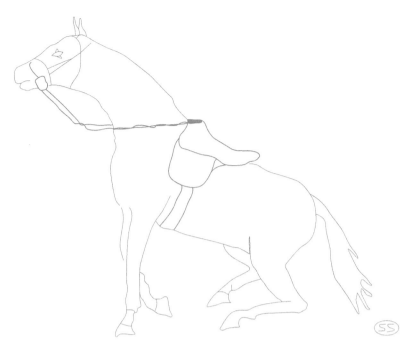

Fig. 3.31. A 'sinking' or 'dipping' action may be seen in a cold-backed horse when mounted.

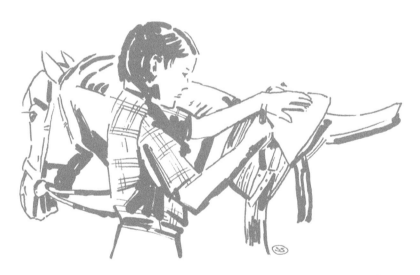

Fig. 3.32. Girthing problems may induce a horse to bite at the handler, or even at the girth itself.

that 89% of horses tested for girthing problems had clinical issues, and 92% of those were gastroscoped and found to have ulcers (Millares-Ramirez and Le Jeune, 2019). There appears, therefore, to be a need to examine any 'girthy' horses for the presence of ulcers and then to treat them, but the condition appears to persist even when horses are considered clear of ulcers. This can be a real problem for owners, particularly as the procedure to investigate ulceration is invasive and expensive, and decisions between the vet and owner must be made in these cases.

SADDLE PADS. Saddles need to be fitted correctly to each individual horse to eliminate pain and pressure problems that might lead to the display of behaviours such as bucking. It is always advisable to first check the saddle of any horse that starts bucking (this behaviour is explained in more detail in Chapter 4). Another factor that is often bypassed by owners and handlers is the various saddle cloths and numnahs available, and the various claims made by different manufacturers. Research has been conducted on the pressure effects of various saddle cloths and in one study it was found that the type of material that gave the most relief from pressure was reindeer fur (Kotschwar *et al.*, 2010). Perhaps this could be related to the use of a sheepskin pad, although to date no research has been conducted comparing the two. Various other designs and padding exist, and choice for the rider is probably made using several different factors such as brand name, attractiveness and claims of efficacy. As research is so scant it is proving rather difficult to isolate the best saddle pad for the greatest effect on performance and behaviour. The other combinations often used under saddles are the numerous types of wedges, saddle risers, gel pads and other items. Again, there is very little research and the rider is left to judge them on their own experiences.

TREELESS SADDLES. There are more complications for riders when deciding what particular saddle suits their horse best and again the choice is huge, with very little research to suggest what the choice should be. It certainly seems that the treeless saddle, once very much in fashion, is not now the first choice of anyone looking to improve their horse's welfare. Removing the tree may seem to give a softer, less restrictive structure for the horse to wear, but studies report that the tree actually disperses the pressure of rider and saddle significantly better and in a superior area compared with the treeless type (Latif *et al.*, 2010; Belock *et al.*, 2012) (Fig. 3.33). Having a tree as part of a saddle also avoids small points of force focus and spreads them out in a way that the treeless saddle does not (Fig. 3.34). If a horse is having a problem with its back, it is well worth trying a correctly fitted treed saddle if the owner has been using a treeless one.

Key points

- Care must be taken in the choice of bit and/or bridle – it is wise to take professional advice if you are not sure or have problems bitting.
- Saddles need to be professionally fitted to avoid causing any problem behaviours related to pain or pressure.
- Be careful in using bitless bridles and treeless saddles, as research to date is debatable regarding their use.
- Many problems can be avoided by thorough and attentive foundation training.

Take-home message

Make sure all tack used is suitable for the horse – and with bits in particular look for solutions to any communication problems before resorting to a stronger bit or novel bridles/nosebands.

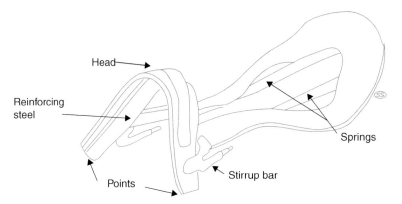

Fig. 3.33. A tree extracted from a saddle showing its ability to spread weight across the horse's back while avoiding the spinal processes.

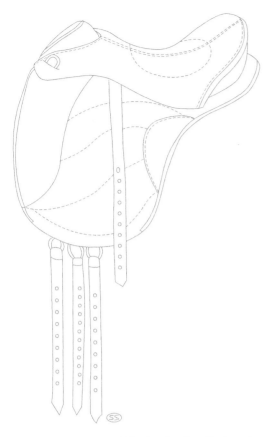

Fig. 3.34. A treeless saddle showing the attachment of stirrup and girth straps – the stirrup placement concentrates pressure on the middle of the saddle pad and the spinal processes.

Case study 1: bitless bridle

An ex-racehorse was the subject of a local visit where the owner had decided to try him in a cross-under bitless bridle to see if it improved his schooling. The call was not directly related to the bitless bridle, but was because the horse had begun to stop when schooling and on hacks. The owner was sympathetic to the horse, having experience in owning ex-racehorses, and so had not put the horse into any situation where it was going to react badly. The horse was observed and seen to stop for no reason that could be detected. If asked to go forwards, the horse would display signs of conflict, including a swishing tail and clamped-back ears. It was then noticed that the horse was wearing a cross-under bridle of the type reported not to release quickly enough for the lack of pressure

to act as a reward, but instead to act as a punishment. It was thought this might possibly explain why the horse had begun to stop: it was not interpreting the correct signal from the rider, due to the lack of pressure-release. The horse was tried in its previous bitted bridle, but it appeared that the problem persisted once the pressure was able to be released, so a programme of retraining was put in place. It was agreed that the horse should use its previous bridle and should stop schooling at present, only being ridden on hacks with other horses, where the motivation to go forwards would be at a premium. The horse would be encouraged to lead the ride; it would be asked to stop correctly by making sure the pressure was released when it started to slow down, and then slowly it would extinguish the learnt behaviour of stopping it had developed.

Another phenomenon that emerged with this horse in its training programme was sensitivity to any signals from the leg or a tap with the whip to encourage forward movement. The horse seemed to react very badly to any pressure from behind the saddle, and the rider assured the behaviourist that they had not put the horse under any undue pressure with either artificial or natural aids. There seemed to be no behavioural or other explanation for this behaviour, so it was suggested to use only light pressure behind the saddle, and use more vocal commands coupled with the use of the ends of the reins as a light touch on either side of the withers. For some reason this worked perfectly and removed the tension reaction of laid-back ears from the horse immediately. This case study really illustrates the fact that strange occurrences with behaviours can happen, and again it is well worth thinking of other methods to use when the usual one fails in its ability to lessen the stress placed on the horse.

Case study 2: girth

This call-out was to a young filly that in its foundation training had developed a real aversion to the girth being fastened up. The training had taken place correctly, with systematic desensitization, and the horse had been turned away for the winter and brought back into work in the early spring. The aversion began when the horse was tacked up for the first time after her period of turn-out, and the behavioural reactions were so strong that the owner became extremely worried. The vet was called out to check over the horse, and it was deemed to be in good health with no visible problems. The vet advised that it was probably not due to ulceration, as the horse had been turned out in a field with companionship and with ad lib haylage provided. Therefore, a solution needed to be devised that was workable for the owner and one that did not place undue stress on the young animal.

The horse was well trained in leading, and as it was led around an indoor school, using counter-conditioning to keep its mind elsewhere, a roller was placed on its back just behind the withers. Following the horse as it was backed up and asked to go forward, the roller leathers were slipped into the buckles and slowly tightened. There were a few behavioural signs of stress, but the filly carried on listening to the handler while the roller was tightened a little more (Fig. 3.35). Once it was secure, the handler led the horse forward and around the school, asking it to stop occasionally, and back up and move to each side. The roller was released after about 10 minutes of leading, and then tightened again with no reaction from the horse. This exercise was repeated five times over the next week, when there was no reaction at all on the final time and the saddle was put in its place. This use of counter-conditioning was not an easy task for the handlers, but with patience and correction the method worked extremely well and rather quickly with little stress to the horse.

Case study 3: bitting

One case involving the use of bits demonstrated how riders can regress to using stronger bits to control their horses, which become more 'dead to the hand' as negative reinforcement is not used correctly and pressure is not released when the horse slows. The horse is not rewarded for slowing, so does not learn that this is what the rider wants, and becomes more and more uncontrollable. This particular horse was a large warmblood, with plenty of muscle and in a rather fit condition. The animal had already been examined for any tooth problems, and also the saddler had inspected its saddle, as these were first considerations for the experienced rider in this case. The rider was now using a gag bit, which acts to pull the horse's head upwards, believed to slow the horse by raising its head under strong pressure. After observing the horse in the arena, it was very plain to see that the rider was having real difficulty in slowing down even in trot, and the horse was showing signs of conflict behaviour with plenty of tail swishing and major ear movements. The rider reported they had used this method of increasing bit strength on several occasions and it had always worked well, but this particular horse had not responded. As the horse was visibly getting increasingly stressed, the session was brought to an end and the rider was asked to walk the horse on a long rein around the school.

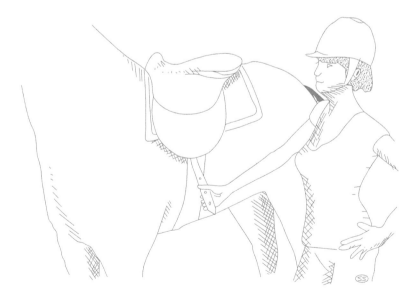

Fig. 3.35. Girth straps held loosely while the pony was led around helped to desensitize the animal in this case.

This showed an interesting development: the horse was perfectly happy to slow and stop once the pressure was removed and the situation de-escalated. The rider was asked to pick up the reins again but without a contact, and surprisingly the horse slowed and stopped without undue stress in walk, and also in a slow trot. As soon as the rider unconsciously asked the horse for a contact it again threw its head up and the rider began to lose control and repeat what had already happened. The problem appeared to be with the pressure from the bit, and as it was known there were no issues with teeth or mouth, it was decided that there was an issue around retraining the horse to accept softer pressure with the use of very accurate negative reinforcement. The rider knew about pressure-release, but was not sure at this stage if they were quite accurate enough with the reward of taking away the aversive pressure when the horse responded by slowing down. It was suggested that the horse should be ridden in just a headcollar with attached reins to completely remove any pressure in its mouth, and also to have a programme of leading, particularly concentrating on getting the 'stop' trained with the least amount of pressure possible. The training was put in place and the rider reported back after a week that they could trot and canter in the school with little pressure applied, and the horse was visibly more relaxed.

A second call-out was made to see how the pair were progressing, and to suggest that the rider should now try a mild snaffle bit while the horse was being observed. Again the horse was not put under any undue stress, and the rider calmly rode around at a walk, asking the horse to stop and start with very light pressure. Soon they progressed to a trot, and again the rider asked lightly and accurately for the halt, before advancing to half-halts, with the halt and leg pressure a split second apart so as not to confuse the horse with a double contradictory signal. On a third visit, the rider was again able to ride the horse in a contact, still using the mild snaffle, but with none of the conflict behaviour that had happened before. The rider did report at a later date that they were using a slightly stronger snaffle for competing, but reverted to using the mild snaffle when schooling and training. It was thought-provoking to see that even this very experienced rider had been having problems with a situation they had always dealt with successfully in the past, but luckily for this horse they were willing to try out a programme of retraining based on equitation science.

Lungeing

One of the fundamentals of foundation training is lungeing, where the horse is trained to move forward in a circle around the handler, signalled by a lengthy rope called a lunge line, the handler's voice and a long lunge whip (Fig. 3.36). Horses are trained to lunge as a precursor to ridden work, to enable them to habituate to the control of their paces and to stop and start signals. A horse can start lunge training with a helper walking the horse on a lead rope around the handler as they ask for the horse to speed up and slow down, using the position of their body and the whip to make a triangle incorporating the horse as the outside edge. By careful positioning of the body and the lunge line, horses will readily learn to stay out on the circle, and move at faster or slower paces as required.

Once the horse is lungeing controllably, a rider is sometimes introduced so that the handler can slowly collate their signals with the rider and the horse learns by classical conditioning that pressure of the legs on their flanks correlates with the pressure from the whip. Care must be taken to match signals, release pressure and make sure signals are consistent to produce a horse that will be ready to leave the lunge line and understand what the rider then wants. Later in their career, lungeing is commonly used to examine lameness and to exercise horses when riding is not possible, for example time constraints, bad weather or dark evenings preventing hacking. Some riders also use lungeing to calm an excitable horse, or give them confidence to ride a horse that maybe has issues such as a cold back. There is no evidence to suggest that any of these methods work and so they are not necessarily recommended for any of these reasons. In addition to this, the use of lungeing to examine lameness may have its problems, as research into lungeing investigating asymmetry has reported that horses that are clinically sound can present as lame when lunged, which means that investigating soundness in this way may have its problems (Rhodin *et al.*, 2016).

Lungeing as a method to retrain horses

More research is needed to confirm how lungeing affects horses before it can be recommended for any type of retraining, mainly due to the appearance and similarity of the method to round-pen training (see earlier). There are similarities seen

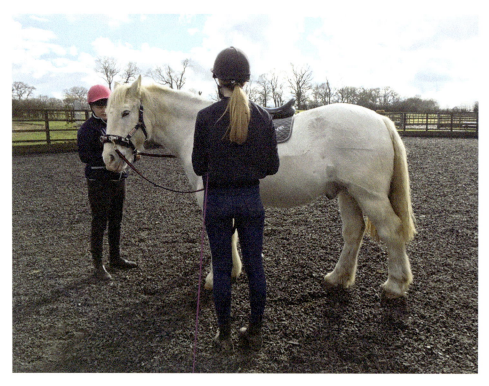

Fig. 3.36. Preparing to lunge a pony with a helper.

between the two, where the horse is encouraged into faster gaits, and this raises cause for concern, because in any other technique for dealing with behavioural problems it is always suggested to slow horses down. This is due to their innate need, as a prey animal, to run to escape aversive situations and it is possible that lungeing, if not carried out in a calm manner, may act to hardwire this avoidance behaviour and make it more likely. Certainly, horses can be retrained to accept natural aids such as voice commands by using the combined lungeing methods and classical conditioning, but there is a question as to whether long-reining is a better system (see below). Also, training aids and gadgets such as those that affect the carriage of the horse are sometimes recommended for rehabilitation and retraining, and these are discussed later in their own section.

Key points

- There is possibly not enough research on the behavioural effects of lungeing on the horse to recommend it as a method for retraining.

- Similarities between lungeing and round-pen training raise questions as to the efficacy of this method for treatment of behavioural problems.
- Lungeing is an extremely popular choice for foundation training and exercise, so must be further examined.

Take-home message

There is a genuine need for research into the behavioural effects of lungeing for use with the horse in foundation training, exercise and retraining.

Case study

The pony involved was engaged in a foundation training programme, and the handler wanted to include lungeing into its repertoire to increase its final sale price. As many people with horses like to lunge for the reasons stated above, it was pertinent to make sure the pony was fully trained in this method. In this case, lungeing training had begun after some groundwork, but the experienced handler was having problems with the pony staying on the outside of the circle and had tried all the techniques he had been using in the past. On arrival, it was observed that the pony seemed uncomfortable on the circle, and kept coming in to the handler off the loop. This appeared to be enough reason to check the pony's physical state and make sure there were no issues regarding lameness or back pain that might be affecting its ability to stay on a circle. Once this was done, and the pony given a full examination, it was revisited and a protocol put in place to retrain the animal to lunge correctly.

The handler was asked to put the pony on to a circle but to then take it off the circle and into a straight line and continue lungeing it down the long side of the school. Once the handler was approaching the corner, the pony was then asked to circle but only until the next long side, where it was instructed to again take a straight line (Fig. 3.37). Permitting the pony to travel in straight lines helped its balance, and as it built its muscles the handler could increase the circling motion until the pony was lungeing freely. What appeared to be a behavioural problem in this case seemed to be purely a lack of balance and development, and after giving the pony the time to build muscle and gain its balance in a natural and uninhibited way the lungeing aspect of circling became a simpler movement for it to make.

Long-reining

The useful practice of long-reining is sometimes part of foundation training but not always, possibly due to the extra exercise the handler has to take part in. Horses are long-reined by wearing their normal bridle, or a lunge cavesson, with two lunge lines attached to each side of the bit rings and then either threaded through the stirrups, if the horse is wearing a saddle, or the roller, or just loose at the horse's flanks. The handler walks behind the horse, signalling it to move much like riding, with the lines used as leg aids (agitating the left lunge line to move right and vice versa) and the hands acting on the lines as reins (Fig. 3.38). The aid to move forward is the vibration of both lines, and the use of vocalization. It must be remembered that the signals need to be stopped immediately the horse begins the movement asked for, to enable negative reinforcement to occur with the removal of pressure. Long-reining should always be started in an enclosed area until the horse learns the signals, and a person to lead the horse at first can help in some circumstances.

Once the horse is proficient and responding to signals well, the handler has the opportunity to long-rein it around fields, on tracks and also perhaps its first experience of the road; however, this is best done in company first and possibly with another person ready to lead the horse if any novel conditions are experienced. Horses will often respond very well to long-reining in this manner, and at the same time the signals being given (on the flanks and with the bit) mimic the reins and legs far better than lungeing seems to. It is also a sound idea to add movements to the training programme, such as weaving in and out of cones to improve responses, 'parking' in coned-off areas, practising backing-up and even going over poles on the ground. This will add some interest to the horse's training programme, and older horses also can benefit from long-reining as a change to their daily lives (Fig. 3.39).

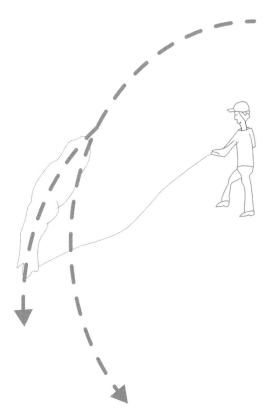

Fig. 3.37. Asking the horse to come off the lungeing circle and walk in a straight line.

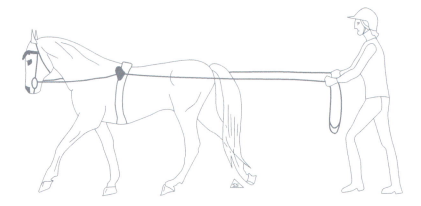

Fig. 3.38. Handlers must be prepared to use negative reinforcement correctly when long-reining a horse, so close attention is needed at all times to make sure pressure is released once the horse walks forward, and is withdrawn when it stops.

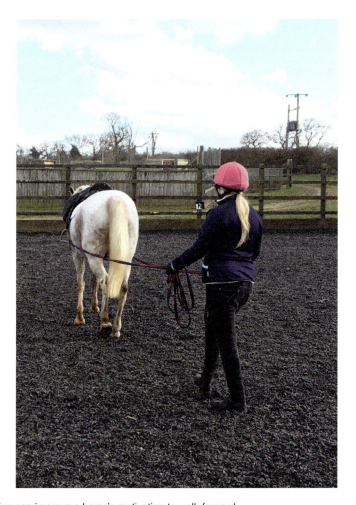

Fig. 3.39. Long-reining can improve a horse's motivation to walk forward.

To date there is no published research concerning long-reining and its use as a method in foundation training or retraining. However, due to the similarity of signals used compared with riding it is possible that the technique is of great benefit to the horse in all stages of its life (Fig. 3.40), and there is certainly a need for research to be undertaken with this system of training.

Key points

- As long-reining is thought to mimic the rider's signals it may be a better way to introduce these signals to the horse rather than lungeing.
- Long-reining appears to be a useful tool to introduce young horses to novel situations, and can be the starter activity for habituating to hacking on the roads.
- There is a pressing need for research in this area.

Take-home message

Perhaps try long-reining with a young horse to replace, or as an addition to, lungeing – it does not have the connotations of lungeing's similarity to round-pen and may systematically train the horse to habituate to a rider's signals in a healthier approach.

Case study

An ex-racehorse was having problems with pigs on a bridle path that the owner wanted to ride on as it led to a wooded area excellent for off-road riding. Various methods had been tried, but the horse either refused to go anywhere near the pigs, or had reared up with another rider and on one occasion bolted off when being led (Fig. 3.41). Another technique was demanded, and long-reining was suggested as a way to progress for this fearful horse. The method of long-reining was one the horse had experienced in the past, and certainly the owner had used it as part of the horse's initial retraining, so a short period of familiarization with the technique was started. Once the horse was responding well to the signals and moving forward freely, the owner began to introduce changes of pace in walk, slowing, stopping and speeding up to improve the lightness of the contact. The overshadowing effect of this type of technical long-reining was hopefully going to act as the catalyst for fear of the pigs to diminish enough that the owner could ride along to the woods without stress.

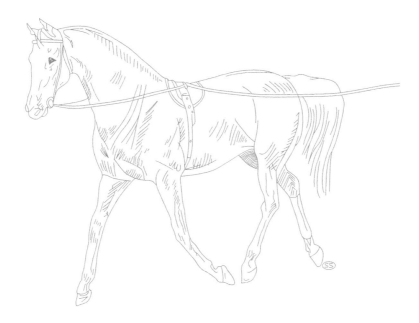

Fig. 3.40. Using the rings higher up on the roller can help to mimic the position of the reins.

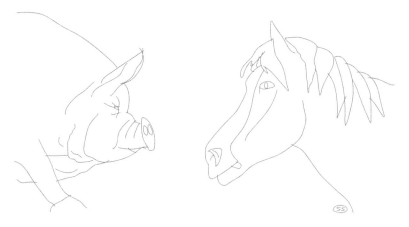

Fig. 3.41. Pigs and horses tend not to get along very well.

The first approach to the pigs was made on a calm, quiet day very early in the morning to avoid most regular dog walkers and runners and to give the horse plenty of space on the shared path. Long-reining began, and on the way to the pigs the handler asked the horse to perform the previous movements in walk of slowing, stopping and speeding up the pace. As the pair advanced towards the problem area the horse did show signs of stress, but not as violent as before, and the handler gave it plenty of time to stop, stand still and move forward slowly as its behaviour dictated. The progress past the pigs took quite a while, but with no real adverse reaction and the horse appeared to be concentrating mostly on the trained movements. In this style the pair managed to pass the pigs and carry on up the track for a way before turning and approaching from the other angle.

The long-reining retraining protocol took place a few times a week, with the owner also incorporating riding at the same time, but not towards the pigs. After a couple of weeks, the owner decided the horse was showing enough improvement to ride past the animals and this was completed successfully the first time, but also with the slowing and speeding up of pace still including overshadowing to some extent. Progressive changes took place and it was not long before the pair were able to ride past the pigs without any undue stress, although the owner reported that they still had to be vigilant of the horse's mood and be ready to use the technique again from the ridden position. This thought-provoking case study illustrates the usefulness of overshadowing in many diverse circumstances with varying retraining needs.

Loading

One of the most common problems for horse owners is issues with loading into trailers for transport. It has been reported that 20% of owners have experienced problems with loading (Yngvesson *et al.*, 2016). It is beneficial to have horses trained to load without any problems, in case of emergencies and trips to the veterinary hospital, rather than having to struggle to get the animal in the trailer when needed. There are various methods to deal with horses that are difficult to load, but the same environmental protocols are useful to follow. These include opening the trailer at the front, perhaps including the front ramp and jockey door to lighten the interior as much as possible, and making sure the angle of the ramp is as low as possible. This can be done by loading on a slight incline, but making sure the trailer is secure when retraining the horse. It is always favourable to have helpers available if needed and for all personnel to be wearing personal protective equipment (PPE).

One of the methods for loading horses is attributed to research into positive reinforcement, where the horse that has the loading problem is first trained to touch a specified target, normally an item like a tennis ball on a short pole (Fig. 3.42). Using operant conditioning with an appetitive reward, horses can be trained very quickly to 'nose-target' and touch a particular object when it is presented to them, and to follow it if it is moved away from them. Once horses having problems with loading are trained to follow the target, it has been reported that they will follow it into the

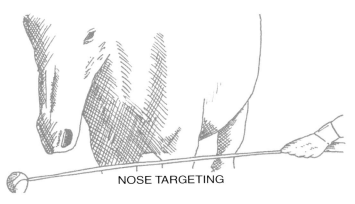

NOSE TARGETING

Fig. 3.42. Target training, or nose-targeting, is a useful method using positive reinforcement.

trailer (Ferguson and Rosales-Ruiz, 2001) and research showed that five mares, who had been loaded with force before, readily learnt the procedure and entered the trailer without hesitation. Another aspect of this research revealed that the mares were able to generalize their learning and also load with a different trailer and handler. The use of negative reinforcement in training methods does seem to reduce stress in already stressed horses, so this method using positive reinforcement may not be best for highly-strung animals (Valenchon *et al.*, 2017).

Leading training can be a useful addition to the behaviourist's tool kit with those more stressful horses that have problems loading. Once the horse has had extensive groundwork applied with clear negative reinforcement signals for go, stop and back, they can be led on to the trailer when in the middle of a training session (Fig. 3.43). If any resistance is encountered, the horse must be kept moving and not stopped for any length of time by the ramp but turned away and approach again. It has been stated anecdotally that 'letting' a horse back off from the ramp is 'teaching' it to do this, but this does not apply if signals are given correctly and the horse is circled, with stop and go signals, and asked to approach the ramp again. Clearly this should be part of a training programme, as with target training, and not used as a method to enable handlers to load the horse at the time it is needed to travel (Fig. 3.44). Like any training, there must be a properly scheduled strategy to follow up to the time the horse needs to load correctly.

Another method to investigate for those horses terrified of the trailer is habituation, where results in these cases have preceded further training such

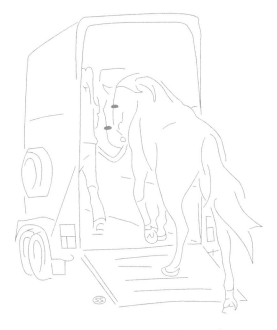

Fig. 3.43. A horse leading correctly into a trailer.

as using a target and correct leading. The horse that is experiencing real fear of the trailer, for whatever reason, will possibly be unable to cope with any technique of loading until its basic fear of the trailer has reduced. Habituation, where an animal is familiarized with an aversive object or situation, is extremely useful in these cases and can enable the next level of training to take place once the fear is extinguished. The knowledge of a distressing experience that the horse retains will slowly reduce as the animal learns that the experience or object does not merit any reaction, and that

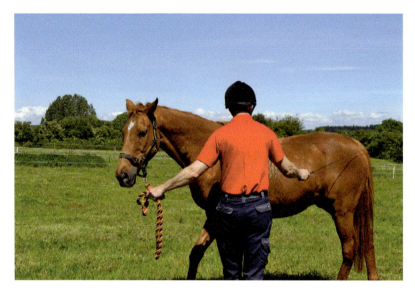

Fig. 3.44. When retraining for loading into a trailer it can sometimes be helpful to make sure the horse's lateral movement in hand is very accurate, as the handler needs control over the direction the horse is walking when entering the trailer and leaving it. This can be accomplished by using a long schooling whip with negative reinforcement and small taps to encourage the lateral movement.

it is not worth its valuable energy to react to it (Christensen *et al.*, 2011).

This process with trailer loading can be undertaken in the simplest way by towing a trailer into the horse's field where the animal is turned out every day, or indeed where it lives out continuously. The horse must be monitored to assess its progress, and once it is beginning to ignore the trailer other techniques such as offering food near or by the trailer can prove useful and help to accelerate the process. When the handler is satisfied with the level of habituation demonstrated by the horse, the other methods such as target training or leading can be utilized.

Key points

- Training a horse to load must be undertaken as a preparation exercise and not when the horse actually needs to be transported.
- Various methods of learning theory can all help to lessen the fear some horses have regarding travelling.
- It is wise to put several procedures in place, such as the wearing of PPE, before attempting any type of training.

Take-home message

Judge the method used on the horse's temperament, and remember the value of taking time with a procedure such as this that can be very aversive to an animal such as the horse that prefers freedom in its surroundings.

Case study

A showjumping Irish warmblood that had been loading well all its life experienced a near catastrophe when travelling to a show. The middle partition of the box it was travelling in with a herd companion came away at the rear of the trailer and was loose in between the two animals (Fig. 3.45). This was only discovered on arrival at the show, and the horses unloaded without showing any outward signs of discomfort. The horse was inspected by the show vet, and no injuries or lameness seemed to have occurred. At the end of the day, as possibly expected, the horse would not load into the trailer and had to be coerced on with lunge lines so that it could be transported back home.

Obviously, a solution had to be sought, as the horse would go to shows on a regular basis, and needed to load and unload without any hesitation

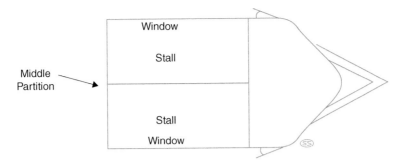

Fig. 3.45. Position of the middle partition in a trailer.

to avoid stress if it was to perform well. It did not seem concerned about the trailer itself, just actually progressing on to the ramp and inside. After the horse had been observed it was noted to be displaying no stress indicators at all; it had decided that whatever aversive methods were used it was not going on to the ramp and would stand quite still, even resting a leg, but not moving forward. The usual techniques were possibly not going to work with this large warmblood, so the owner was asked about the horse's temperament and if there was anything that was particularly appetitive for it. Questioning owners is often very profitable and in this case study the horse was described as very motivated towards food, particularly soaked sugar beet, so a proposal was devised to help the owner successfully load their horse again.

The trailer was moved into the owner's yard from the car park area so it was easily accessible to them. It was secured safely and in a place with plenty of room for movement for the horse so that it did not instigate feelings of pressure for it to step up on to the ramp. The protocol decided upon was explained to the owner, who then followed a plan of feeding the horse its usual ration in the same yellow bucket twice a day but placing it nearer and nearer the ramp. After a week the horse was stepping up on to the ramp to eat its feeds, and then exiting by the front ramp without the breast bar in place (Fig. 3.46). Another week saw it eating quietly in the trailer itself. Next, the ramp was lifted into place when the horse was eating, and this progressed to the owner putting up the ramp, going in through the jockey door and leading the horse out instead of letting it exit by itself. By this time the horse was relaxed enough to be led into the trailer, eat a few treats given to it by the owner, and depart down the front ramp. Thus, a very

complicated situation was solved with no pressure or aversive action, and the horse stayed unstressed throughout the whole procedure. However, it is important to note in the situation explained above that the horse was of a calm temperament and did not in any way give the impression of being fearful of the trailer. This method may not necessarily work with a horse of different attitude, and other, more controlled protocols such as target training would be better used in this circumstance.

Coping with events and competitions

Foundation training usually involves exposure to various novel circumstances for most horses, and first events are dealt with in the same way – smaller shows at first, where the horse may just go to watch, or walk around, progressing to entering in small classes. Many horses habituate in this way extremely well and start to generalize with more and more shows attended. Each aspect, such as clapping, larger audiences and maybe discipline-specific unique situations such as new jump types or potted plants at dressage, can all be dealt with at home first if needed (Fig. 3.47). Occasionally horses can show signs of stress with certain environments, but many experienced trainers will make sure that any exposure is attempted firstly at home, for instance with a starting bell. If there is a known stressor, this can be dealt with singly, either by exposure with desensitization if the case allows, or by habituation if the issue is with inanimate objects, by placing them in the home setting. Other situations may call for more detailed planning and interaction if the horse is really disturbed by the circumstance.

Overshadowing is a useful tool for the behaviourist in many of these experiences, where the handler or owner probably would already lead their trained horse around on foot at first to allow it to adapt to novel

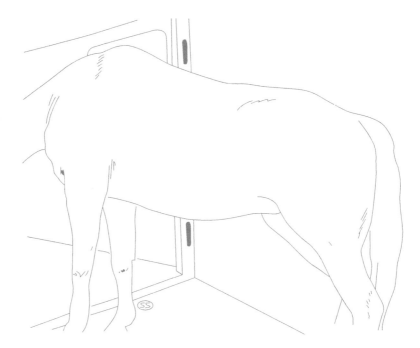

Fig. 3.46. A horse gradually stepping on to the ramp of a trailer with the incentive of food.

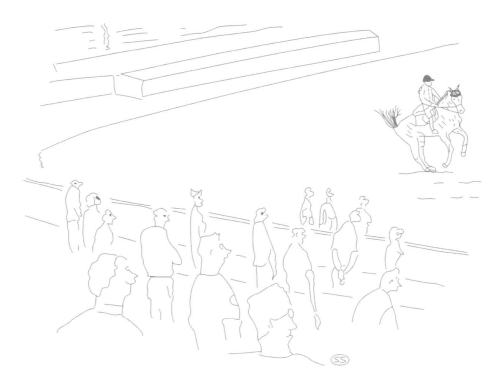

Fig. 3.47. Horses need to be habituated to crowds of people and can be desensitized by travelling to smaller shows and progressing to larger events.

occurrences at an event showground. However, for a well-trained horse responding to leading exercises as stipulated previously, this method could be used at any point, to bring the attention back to the handler. For example, if the horse is becoming very excited at the presence of so many different horses, a short period of leading forwards and reversing along with lateral movement tends to act as a catalyst for overshadowing as the horse concentrates on its training and slowly beings to adapt to the environment it is in.

Counter-conditioning could work extremely well with a horse that is fearful of particular aspects of events, such as a real fear of the sound of a loudspeaker (Fig. 3.48). It is common to play radios or recordings to horses and other animals to allay their fear of certain sounds, first quietly and then building in volume, but sound systems are quite a different factor, due to their loudness and unexpectedness. The case study below exemplifies one such learning process.

Key points

- Many methods can be used to habituate horses to events and competitions, and often a combination is used by handlers.
- If a horse experiences an aversive event, it is possible that it may need tailored retraining to overcome the unpleasant memories of it.
- Foundation training should ideally incorporate travel to events; local shows provide perfect opportunities for this as a starter exercise.

Fig. 3.48. Loud noises, such as loud speakers and sound systems, can be very aversive to horses.

Take-home message

No horse will ever be fully prepared for their first show, but if the horse has an established level of foundation training this will make dealing with any situation that may occur easier.

Case study

This horse was a veteran of shows but had not gone to any for quite a period of time and the owner wanted to take it again to start doing some veteran showing. The first show had a sound system that was extremely loud, and the horse was quite incapable of coping with the volume of noise. It was not the only one, as a few owners complained, but in this case the horse was already very fearful and at one point had bolted away from the owner. Back at home again the owner asked for help in retraining the horse to cope with the loud sound systems now commonly being used at shows. The horse was visited to gain an impression of its temperament and observe its actions when a recording of a speaker system was played. The reaction was very pronounced, so a simple programme of retraining was put in place with the owner's help. The programme contained a measure of counter-conditioning, where the owner was asked to feed the horse while the recording of the sound system was playing. To enable counter-conditioning to take place, It was very important to make sure that the horse was fed at exactly the time the recording was played.

The programme was repeated for a couple of weeks, then the horse went to its first show where there was a loudspeaker system set up. The owner reported back that the horse experienced no problems whatsoever and appeared to ignore the sound system rather than look for food. Back at home the horse now had its feed without any recordings, and the owner never experienced problems again at shows with speaker systems.

References

Belock, I.B., Kaiser, J., Lavagnino, M. and Clayton, H.M. (2012) Comparison of pressure distribution under a conventional saddle and a treeless saddle at sitting trot. *The Veterinary Journal* 193(1), 87–91.

Bjornsdottir, S., Frey, R., Kristjansson, T. and Lundstrom, T. (2014) Bit-related lesions in Icelandic competition horses. *Acta Veterinaria Scandinavica* 56(1), 40.

Christensen, J.W. (2013) Object habituation in horses: the effect of voluntary versus negatively reinforced approach to frightening stimuli. *Equine Veterinary Journal* 45(3), 298–301.

Christensen, J.W. (2016) Early-life object exposure with a habituated mother reduces fear reactions in foals. *Animal Cognition* 19(1), 171–179.

Christensen, J.W., Zharkikh, T. and Chovaux, E. (2011) Object recognition and generalisation during habituation in horses. *Applied Animal Behavioural Science* 129(2–4), 83–91.

Cook, W.R. and Mills, D.S. (2009) Preliminary study of jointed snaffle vs. cross-under bitless bridles: quantified comparison of behaviour in four horses. *Equine Veterinary Journal* 41(8), 827–830.

Crago, F., Shea, G., James, O., Schemann, K. and McGreevy, P.D. (2019). An opportunistic pilot study of radiographs of equine nasal bones at the usual site of nosebands. *Journal of Veterinary Behaviour* 29, 70–76.

Cross, G.H., Cheung, M.K.P., Honey, T.J., Pau, M.K. and Senior, K.-J. (2017). Application of a dual force sensor system to characterize the intrinsic operation of horse bridles and bits. *Journal of Equine Veterinary Science* 48, 129–135.

De Cocq, P., Van Weeren, P.R. and Back, W. (2004) Effects of girth, saddle and weight on movements of the horse. *Equine Veterinary Journal* 36(8), 758–763.

Doherty, O., Casey, V., McGreevy, P., McLean, A., Parker, P. and Arkins, S. (2017a) An analysis of visible patterns of horse bit wear. *Journal of Veterinary Behavior* 18, 84–91.

Doherty, O., Conway, T., Conway, R., Murray, G. and Casey, V. (2017b) An objective measure of noseband tightness and its measurement using a novel digital tightness gauge. *PLoS ONE* 12(1), e0168996.

Fédération Equestre International (2020) Dressage Rules. Available at: https://inside.fei.org/system/files/16.3_ANNEX_GA19_DRESSAGE%20RULES.pdf (accessed 19 May 2020).

Fenner, K., Yoon, S., White, P., Starling, M. and McGreevy, P. (2016) The effect of noseband tightening on horses' behavior, eye temperature, and cardiac responses. *PLoS ONE* 11(5), e0154179.

Fenner, K., McLean, A.N. and McGreevy, P.D. (2019). Cutting to the chase: How round-pen, lunging and high-speed liberty work may compromise horse welfare. *Journal of Veterinary Behaviour* 29, 88–94.

Ferguson, D.L. and Rosales-Ruiz, J. (2001) Loading the problem loader: the effects of target training and shaping on trailer-loading behavior of horses. *Journal of Applied Behavior Analysis* 34(4), 409–423.

Henshall, C. and McGreevy, P.D. (2014) The role of ethology in round-pen horse training – a review. *Applied Animal Behavior* 155, 1–11.

Hockenhull, J. and Creighton, E. (2012) Equipment and training risk factors associated with ridden behaviour problems in UK leisure horses. *Applied Animal Behaviour Science* 137(1-2), 36–42.

Ijichi, C., Tunstall, S., Putt, E. and Squibb, K. (2018) Dually noted: the effects of a pressure headcollar on compliance, discomfort and stress in horses during handling. *Applied Animal Behaviour* 205, 68–73.

Kienapfel, K., Link, Y. and Konig von Borstel, U. (2014) Prevalence of different head–neck positions in horses shown at dressage competitions and their relation to conflict behaviour and performance marks. *PLoS ONE* 9(8), e103140.

Kotschwar, A.B., Baltacis, A. and Peham, C. (2010) The effects of different saddle pads on forces and pressure distribution beneath a fitting saddle. *Equine Veterinary Journal* 42(2), 114–118.

Krueger, K. (2007) Behaviour of horses in the 'round-pen technique'. *Applied Animal Behaviour Science* 104(1-2), 162–170.

Kydd, E., Padalino, B., Henshall, C. and McGreevy, P. (2017) An analysis of equine round-pen training videos posted online: differences between amateur and professional trainers. *PLoS ONE* 12(9), e0184851.

Lashley, M., Nauwelaerts, S., Vernooij, J., Back, W. and Clayton, H.M. (2014) Comparison of the head and neck position of elite dressage horses during top-level competitions in 1992 versus 2008. *Veterinary Journal* 202(3), 462–465.

Latif, S.N., von Peinen, K., Wiestner, T., Bitschau, C., Renk, B. and Weishaupt, M.A. (2010) Saddle pressure patterns of three different training saddles (normal tree, flexible tree, treeless) in Thoroughbred racehorses on trot and gallop. *Equine Veterinary Journal* 42(s38).

Manfredi, J.M., Rosenstein, D., Lanovaz, J.L., Nauwelaerts, S. and Clayton, H.M. (2009) Fluoroscopic study of oral behaviours in response to the presence of a bit and the effects of rein tension. *Comparative Exercise Physiology* 6(4), 143–148.

Marsboll, A.F. and Christensen, J.W. (2015) Effects of handling on fear reactions in young Icelandic horses. *Equine Veterinary Journal* 47(5), 615–619.

McGreevy, P.D. (2007) The advent of equitation science. *Veterinary Journal* 174, 492–500.

McGreevy, P., Warren-Smith, A. and Guisard, Y. (2012) The effect of double bridles and jaw-clamping crank nosebands on temperature of eyes and facial skin of horses. *Journal of Veterinary Behavior: Clinical Applications and Research* 7(3), 142–148.

McLean, A.N. and McGreevy, P.D. (2010) Horse training techniques that may defy the principles of learning theory and compromise welfare. *Journal of Animal Behaviour* 5, 187–195.

Millares-Ramirez, E.M. and Le Jeune, S.S. (2019) Girthiness: retrospective study of 37 horses (2004–2016). *Journal of Equine Veterinary Science* 79, 100–104.

Murray, R., Guire, R., Fisher, M. and Fairfax, V. (2015) A bridle designed to avoid peak pressure locations under the headpiece and noseband is associated with more uniform pressure and increased carpal and tarsal flexion, compared with the horse's usual bridle.

Journal of Equine Veterinary Science 35(11–12), 947–955.

Rhodin, M., Johnston, C., Holm, K.R., Wennerstrand, J. and Drevemo, S. (2005) The influence of head and neck position on kinematics of the back in riding horses at the walk and trot. *Equine Veterinary Journal* 37, 7–11.

Rhodin, M., Roepstorff, L., French, A., Keegan, K.G., Pfau, T. and Egenvall, A. (2016) Head and pelvic movement asymmetry during lungeing in horses with symmetrical movement on the straight. *Equine Veterinary Journal* 48(3), 315–320.

Scofield, R.M. and Randle, H. (2012) Comparison of behaviour exhibited by horses ridden in conventional bitted and bitless bridles. In: Randle, H., Waran, N. and Williams, J. (eds) *Proceedings of the 8th International Society for Equitation Science Conference* July 2012, Royal (Dick) University, Edinburgh, p. 133.

Scofield, R.M. and Randle, H. (2013) Preliminary comparison of behaviors exhibited by horses ridden in bitted and bitless bridles. *Journal of Veterinary Behaviour: Clinical Applications and Research* 8(2), 20–21.

Tabor, G. and Williams, J. (2018) Equine rehabilitation: a review of trunk and hind limb muscle activity and exercise selection. *Journal of Equine Veterinary Science* 60, 97–103.

Toft, K., Kjeldsen, S.T., Otten, N.D., Galen, G., Fjeldborg, J. *et al.* (2020) Evaluation of dynamic structural disorders in the upper airways and applied rein tension in healthy dressage horses during riding in different gaits and head–neck positions. *Science* 87, 102934.

Uldahl, M. and Clayton, H.M. (2019) Lesions associated with the use of bits, nosebands, spurs and whips in Danish competition horses. *Equine Veterinary Journal* 51(2), 154–162.

Valenchon, M., Levy, F., Moussu, C. and Lansade, L. (2017) Stress affects instrumental learning based on positive or negative reinforcement in interaction with personality in domestic horses. *PLoS ONE* 12(5), e0170783.

Visser, E.K., Kuypers, M.M.F., Stam, J.S.M. and Riedstra, B. (2019) Practice of noseband use and intentions towards behavioural change in Dutch equestrians. *Animals (Basel)* 9(12), e1131.

Von Borstel, U.U., Duncan, I.J.H., Shoveller, A.K., Merkies, K., Keeling, L.J. and Millman, S.T. (2009) Impact of riding in a coercively obtained Rollkur posture on welfare and fear of performance horses. *Applied Animal Behaviour Science* 116, 228–236.

Walker, V.A., Dyson, S.J. and Murray, R.C. (2013) Effect of a Pessoa® training aid on temporal, linear and angular variables of the working trot. *Veterinary Journal* 198(2), 404–11.

Warren-Smith, A.K. and McGreevy, P.D. (2008). Preliminary investigations into the ethological relevance of round-pen (round-yard) training of horses. *Journal of Applied Animal Welfare Science* 11(3), 285–98.

Weishaupt, M.A., Wiestner, T., von Peinen, K., Waldern, N., Roepstorff, L. *et al.* (2006) Effect of head and neck position on vertical ground reaction forces and interlimb coordination in the dressage horse ridden at walk and trot on a treadmill. *Equine Veterinary Journal* 38(36), 387–392.

Wilk, I. and Janczarek, I. (2015) Relationship between behaviour and cardiac response to round-pen training. *Journal of Veterinary Behaviour* 10(3), 231–236.

Yngvesson, J., de Boussard, E.M., Larsson, M. and Lundberg, A. (2016) Loading horses (*Equus caballus*) onto trailers – behaviour of horses and horse owners during loading and habituating. *Applied Animal Behaviour Science* 184, 59–65.

4 Ridden Work

The Phenomenon of the Barefoot Horse – Evidence and Discussion

The increase in the number of horses kept barefoot is a modern occurrence, recorded in 2013 as representing 24% of the equine population of the UK (Hockenhull and Creighton, 2013). Barefoot as a trend was generally brought to the attention of the equine world by purveyors of natural horsemanship, who are attempting to work towards keeping horses in a holistic way. This might include the use of treeless saddles and bitless bridles, with environmental changes such as 24-hour turnout and ad lib fibre, and may also involve discarding the traditional practice of nailing shoes on to hooves. As research develops in this area, the anecdotal reports of barefoot horses competing, particularly in endurance, and also in hacking homes, have become more common and are regularly discussed in the media (Fig. 4.1).

Hoof abnormalities are the commonest factor of lameness in horses as reported by owners (Thirkell and Hyland, 2017), so a move to techniques that may reduce these incidences of lameness is always sought by them. These may include using hoof dressings, trying out various types of remedial shoeing as recommended by professionals, and feeding their horses supplements, but ultimately the search may push owners towards an investigation into the possibility of 'going barefoot'. This conversion appears to be much more challenging than just removing the shoes and letting the horse cope itself. Indeed, the 'transition to barefoot' may encompass a change in environment, diet, a gradual return to work after the shoes have been removed and regular trimming with plenty of recourse to 'trotting-up' at each interval and close examination of the hoof (K. Jay, personal communication, 25 October 2019). Certainly, in recent years there have been relatively more studies into the comparison of shod and barefoot trimmed horses as more owners move to using this method, including professional dressage riders and eventers. Some racehorse stables are trialling barefoot, particularly in rehabilitation, and also some medical conditions such as navicular syndrome have been tested with barefoot trimming.

The idea behind the use of barefoot trimming instead of remedial shoeing has shown its merits in the recent studies examining the changes of hoof morphology when horses are trimmed for barefoot performance instead of being shod (Fig. 4.2). Barefoot trimming employs better usage of the frog, bars and sole of the hoof to bear the horse's weight and has been reported to elevate the heel and increase the solar angle of the pedal bone (Clayton *et al.*, 2011). These beneficial changes to the structure of the hoof and peripheral skeleton appear to reduce underrun heels and also place the pedal bone in a more structurally sound position – both very useful in the treatment of not just navicular syndrome but other conditions and diseases as well (Fig. 4.3). It is known that shoeing reduces the frog's contact with the ground (Bowker, 2003a), increases the mechanical loading of the lower limb (Moyer and Anderson, 1975), and also restricts movement and contraction at the heel (Brunsting *et al.*, 2019). These restrictions of movement and extra loading appear to decrease the size of the hoof to the extent where atrophy could be happening, and coronary band circumference and hoof angle show significant increases in barefoot horses compared with shod horses in only 7 weeks of growth (Malone and Davies, 2019).

Horses' hooves readily adapt to the environment in which they exist (Bowker, 2003b), and those starting the transition to barefoot immediately have increased vascular capacity (blood supply) as soon as the shoes are removed (Gunkelman *et al.*, 2017). A programme of transition must be followed as advised, although anecdotally some horses will make the change to barefoot very quickly. This allows the adaptation of the hooves to hard surfaces such as roads, and research is needed here to

© R. Scofield 2020. *Solving Equine Behaviour Problems* (R. Scofield)

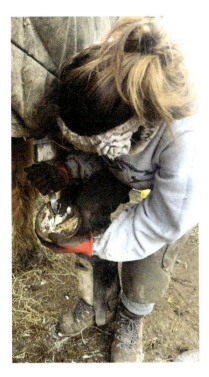

Fig. 4.1. A qualified barefoot trimmer shaping the frog of a horse who suffered from navicular syndrome before treatment.

test how long this takes in various circumstances so that the owner may be informed of the correct timespan. Nevertheless, the effect of increased blood supply to the hooves can be a difficult concept to appreciate, as the traditional advice of feeling for a 'cold leg' in a sound horse and looking for areas of warmth as an indication of problems does not work well in a barefoot horse, where their legs are warm to the touch due to the increased blood supply. This is evidenced when using thermography, and horses that are shod will experience a continual lowering of the temperature of their hooves as they wait for their next shoeing procedure (Gunkelman *et al.*, 2017). The increase of vascularity to the hoof is also demonstrated in the significant increase of the depth of digital cushioning, seen in barefoot horses over a 140-day test period in comparison with shod horses (Proske *et al.*, 2017). Depth of this tissue is very important to the health of the equine hoof, and it appears that the barefoot trim enabling the soles of the hooves rather than the walls to bear weight increases the growth of vascularization enough to remodel the entire hoof over time (Fig. 4.4).

Even if horses are not transitioned to barefoot, the research certainly points towards reducing the period between shoeing as a real consideration if healthy hooves are to be maintained (Malone and Davies, 2019). Regular trimming of the barefoot horse, including the natural reduction of the hoof in contact with the ground, seems to prevent this occurring and enables the hoof to remodel without restriction (Fig. 4.5). As hooves grow continuously, and shoes restrict this growth, the angles of the bones change over shoeing periods to present real changes that may increase the possibility of tendon and ligament failure (Moleman *et al.*, 2006). As toes grow longer in shod feet, gluteal pain can develop (Mansmann *et al.*, 2010) and cause intermittent and often unidentifiable pain. A routine decrease of the 'breakover' point of the hoof, where the stride involves movement of the hoof across the ground to its next position, also reduces stress around the navicular structures (Page and Hagen, 2002), further indicating that shoeing intervals should be as short as is possible. Another very common tradition involves the use of shoes on only the front feet, aiming perhaps to reduce cost for the owner. However, this method is linked to performance problems with the uneven weight distribution affecting, for instance, the jumping ability of the horse and reported to be associated with increased risk of jumping problems (Hockenhull and Creighton, 2012).

Currently there is a growing body of evidence for examining shoeing in its traditional form, and indisputably different methods of shoeing, shorter periods of time between the process and other materials and designs for shoes are being investigated. It is worth remembering that, in an experiment to evaluate the damage inflicted on horse long bones by various shoeing materials in a simulated kick, at an impactor velocity of 8 m per second, the probability of a fracture with a steel-shod hoof was 75%, and that of aluminium shoes was 81%, while plastic shoes and the unshod hoof did not damage the bones (Sprick *et al.*, 2017). An investigation of different shoe shapes looked at a novel metal split-toe shoe in comparison with a traditional shoe and a barefoot trim, with results for the split-toe shoe mimicking closely the barefoot hoof's superior movement and ability for the heel to contract, not seen with the shod hoof (Brunsting *et al.*, 2019). The split-toe shoe is nailed on as normal, but then divided at the toe, appearing to allow lateral movement across the hoof. Plastic, rubber and steel shoes have been examined for any differing capacity in

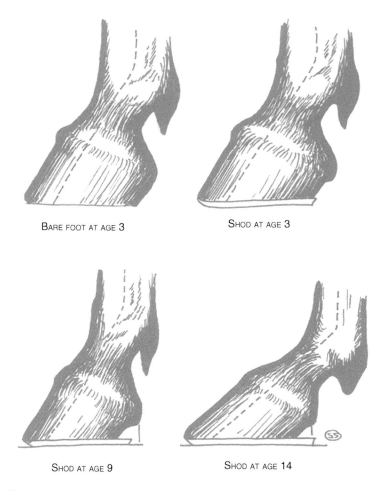

BARE FOOT AT AGE 3   SHOD AT AGE 3

SHOD AT AGE 9   SHOD AT AGE 14

Fig. 4.2. An illustration to demonstrate how the hoof can change over many years of shoeing to become underrun with collapsed heels.

allowing foot slip on concrete (Pardoe *et al.*, 2001), but no significant difference was seen across the varying materials. Foot slip is an important consideration, as the hoof needs to slide slightly on striking the ground to allow dissipation of shearing or cranial-caudal ground reaction forces that can be damaging to tissues. This raises the issue of the use of studs, on the road, on grass and in other circumstances, where a degree of removal of the natural ability to dissipate shearing forces may perhaps be damaging anatomical structures (Harvey *et al.*, 2012). In another development, glue was used to attach plastic shoes rather than nails as used with metal types, perhaps seen as more beneficial to the horse. However, it was reported that this method allows even less heel movement than traditional

shoes (Yoshihara *et al.*, 2010), therefore compounding the inherent problem with the lack of heel contraction and movement in shod horses.

Problems Investigated

Mounting

In its foundation training every horse needs to have some sessions involving standing still while being mounted. This could be at a mounting block, or from the ground, but due to recent research it appears to improve welfare if a mounting block is used by limiting the strain on the horse's back from the action of the weight (and foot) in the stirrup (Geutjens *et al.*, 2008). This is due to stresses apparent on the horse's back whilst mounting is

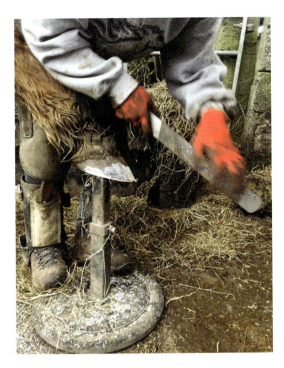

Fig. 4.3. Shaping the outer hoof wall of a horse with navicular syndrome.

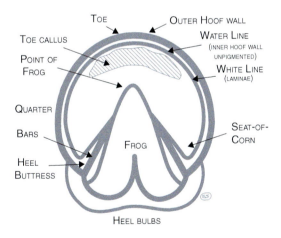

Fig. 4.4. Barefoot hooves are trimmed to allow the sole to come into contact with the ground, and in the transition period they develop 'toe calluses' as seen here.

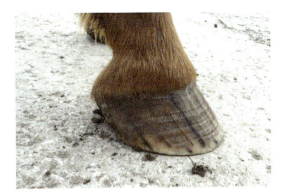

Fig. 4.5. A well-shaped barefoot hoof on a 25-year-old Thoroughbred who presented initially with underrun and collapsed heels.

taking place, where the right-hand side of the wither area is subjected to the highest pressure, seeming to suggest that this significant area of the spinal processes acts to steady the saddle worn by the horse at the time of mounting. If mounting blocks are constructed so that the rider does not actually need to place their foot in the stirrup, but their first action is to swing their leg over the horse's back, then possibly all pressure normally placed on the wither area would reduce drastically. A steadying hand placed on the withers would act as a balance, but there would be no shearing forces from the action of the foot in the stirrup in relation to the withers. It is therefore recommended for owners and riders to investigate the provision of higher mounting blocks, though advised that research to investigate this potential lack of force from very high mounting blocks would be prudent.

It is rewarding if a horse stands still while it is mounted, and also in some situations it can be dangerous to have a horse that will not stand still, such as on a hack, if for any reason the horse needs to be mounted from a wall or gate. Certainly in foundation training the horse must habituate to the presence of a human on its back, and this is normally trained in stages using desensitization where the rider will gradually lean over further and further until they are able to go astride the horse and eventually sit up straight. Once this is accomplished the act of mounting from a block must be incorporated into the training, so this is where a strong basis in groundwork and leading comes into effect, with the horse that is trained to stand still until being asked to move. This should not be any different from the stance of the mounting block, although some horses are bothered by the difference in height and this again can be trained using desensitization.

Problems usually arise with mounting from riders not being conscientious enough to make sure the horse does stand still while at the block, slowly conditioning them to move off before being asked for any number of reasons. It is therefore strongly advised to always act on the protocol of training the horse to stand and not to deviate from this. It may be seen as not particularly problematic if a horse moves off a little quickly, but this can prove disastrous if a rider falls from their mount at any point and needs to remount a possibly rather stimulated animal. There may not be anyone around to help, and a well-trained horse that stands in these circumstances is a valuable asset.

In some cases, horses have been trained to be mounted in differing ways, for instance when racehorses are being mounted. The work riders or jockeys generally have a leg-up from the trainer or stable staff, rather than using a block, to enable the horses to keep warm and moving (Fig. 4.6). This can prove problematic when racehorses find homes after their careers and then need to be trained to stand still,

which can take time; it has not been part of their repertoire for sometimes many years. In these cases, a programme of leading groundwork is highly recommended at first, which can then progress to work while ridden, perhaps with a handler involved if the ex-racehorse is conditioned to move off when being mounted. Another method of retraining the ex-racehorse is covered in the case study below.

Key points

- The act of mounting can affect the welfare of the horse, therefore the use of high mounting blocks is recommended.
- Riders are encouraged to always ask their horse to stand still while being mounted, and not to fall into the habit of letting the horse move off prematurely.

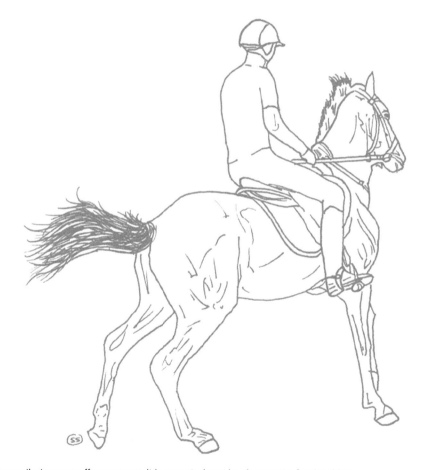

Fig. 4.6. A horse that moves off as soon as it is mounted can be dangerous for the rider.

- Each individual case must be observed and examined; however, it is inevitable that leading training will play a large part in removing undesirable mounting behavioural problems.
- Remember some disciplines such as horseracing may train horses differently – and may not use a mounting block at all.

Take-home message

It is far easier to make mounting a part of a horse's foundation training and to retain the capability of the horse to stand still at a mounting block than to retrain it when problems occur.

Case study

This case study involved an ex-racehorse who had been purchased from the trainer to enter a new life in dressage. The horse in question lacked speed, but was very easy to back in its foundation training, had excellent paces and movement, and had shown a large amount of potential as an animal that would accept retraining into a new discipline. The new owner was prepared to give the horse time to adapt, and once purchased the animal was given a month off before being brought into work again, starting with a programme of leading training. The horse was progressing really well, until the time came to start riding and then problems began with mounting. The owner had tried to integrate the leading training with standing at the mounting block, and this appeared to work extremely well until the rider was waiting on the block to mount. This triggered the horse to revert back to its original training and it would move off straightaway. The owner trialled a handler holding the horse, and using the leading method to ask it to stand, but this only exacerbated matters and the horse always began to get stressed. The horse had its first visit and was observed while the rider tried to mount. A positive reinforcement method using treats was discounted, because the horse seemed very stressed about the whole situation and actually ignored any motivation towards an appetitive reward. This is an unusual circumstance, but not completely unknown, so another method had to be sought.

After the initial observation, the horse was mounted in its usual way and the owner was asked if its back had been checked. Whilst being ridden the horse was calm and displayed no signs of conflict behaviours, and actually worked rather well. A method was devised that was rather unorthodox, but in this case proved to work well. At the outset the horse started a programme of leading training again, though this time including poles on the ground to act as a 'parking space' where the horse was led into, and then backed out. Standing still in the parking space was imperative, and the horse therefore trained to stand for a few minutes while it was being held in the space. This progressed to the utilization of the corner of the school, with one pole, to mimic the parking space but with two solid walls. The horse readily generalized its behaviour to the new protocol and was always backed out of the space, keeping a very straight line walking backwards.

Soon the rider began to take part, firstly in the parking space just with poles, as part of their usual groundwork, but then progressing to the corner of the school. The rider kept the horse straight, moving slowly and asking the animal to stand still once in the space. Once the horse appeared to accept this new movement along with the rest of its training, the behaviourist arranged another visit for the next stage in using the mounting block. The owner was asked to arrange to have a mounting block moved into the school, and then the retraining took place using the parking space with poles at first, only to progress to the corner of the school if needed.

The horse was led to the parking space and the mounting block and stood still as the rider mounted, demonstrating the reinforcing effect of using thorough retraining. The horse was then asked to walk straight out of the parking space once the pole was removed, and then walked around the school. The owner kept the poles in place for a few days, and then dispensed with them altogether, progressing to using the mounting block outside. The ex-racehorse never attempted to move from its original standing position, and the owner was advised to make sure that they asked the horse to stand still until they were mounted, and not to accept any movement. It was an interesting solution, and one that was devised using a mix of learning theories, from generalization to negative reinforcement.

Napping

Napping describes the problem behaviour of a horse not wanting to leave its yard for a hack, or just standing still and refusing to move forwards in any given situation (Fig. 4.7). Any horse presenting with this behaviour should be at first thoroughly

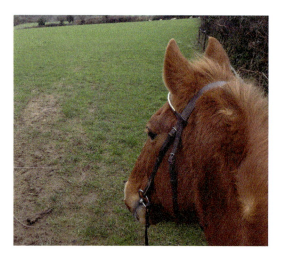

Fig. 4.7. Horses should readily move forward if signalled by their rider.

examined by a vet, as there could well be a degree of low-grade lameness, perhaps in the front feet, that has not been discovered before. Overall, out of a cohort of 3000 purportedly sound sports and leisure horses, 14.5% tested positive for abnormal movement and 4.8% presented were clinically lame (Visser *et al.*, 2014). Indeed, owners reported that 33% of horses under their care had experienced lameness at some point in their working careers (Murray *et al.*, 2010) and there is evidence that more than 47% of the sports horse population in the UK may be lame (Dyson *et al.*, 2018), so lameness is undoubtedly not an uncommon occurrence and deserves to be investigated. Anecdotally, many of the cases of napping visited and then referred for investigation by the vet have then presented with very low-grade lameness issues, and several of these, once examined fully, often confirm the first signs of navicular disease. It is therefore recommended that the horse in question should be tested for lameness and only then to proceed with solving the problem if it is identified as a behaviour issue.

The behaviour of napping is an interesting one, as horses being prey animals favour flight over fight; therefore, not wanting to move forward for whatever reason must have its origin in an intense experience. It is wise also to check for any other health issues, such as the teeth and indeed back, and then the bridle and saddle to make sure everything is fitted correctly and not causing any discomfort. It would appear at this stage to have

eliminated most cases of napping, but some do remain, posing a behavioural issue for owners and handlers, and some changes to the horse's riding practice may bring a quick solution. These might include examining whether the horse is ridden out on its own – is it a young horse, just beginning its hacking experience, or has the horse been moved to a different yard and lost its usual hacking partners? Certainly, one method to combat these situations is for the horse to be ridden out with its herd companions, and this may solve the problem: if the horse is able to follow others and is then asked to take the lead, this may help the horse to learn that it is able to walk at the front without undue stress. This process can take time, and obviously, horses do have different characteristics in their temperaments, so some may always continue to feel safer at the back of a ride or in the middle.

For the horse showing signs of napping in other situations, the reason and origin for this behaviour can sometimes be discovered. For example, a horse may not want to leave its herd companions and walk away from the field, as horses value companionship above most other motivational needs. There may be other environmental causes, and if discovered some measures can be put in place to solve them or routines might be reorganized to better enable the horse to cope with any undesirable circumstances. However, sometimes help is needed to observe behaviour and try to ascertain the aetiology of the reaction, and then decide which is the most practical method of using learning theory to solve the napping problem. Three examples are illustrated in the case studies below, each with different solutions to help overcome this most frustrating of behavioural problems.

Key points

- There are many different reasons for napping, and some may well be linked to low-grade lameness so it is always advised to have a lameness examination by the vet first.
- Also, it is advisable to have the horse's teeth and back checked, along with the fit of its bridle and saddle.
- If the horse is judged sound and in no discomfort, it is time to try to locate the origin and/or reason for the behaviour, and then build a retraining programme from this point.

Take-home message

Any incidence of napping must at first be checked for pain issues, either from lameness, teeth or back problems, and also bridle and saddle fit.

Case study 1

The first case study does not involve riding, but an interesting incidence of a horse going out on loan and then starting to nap when it was led from its stable to the field. The horse was checked for any other limiting factors, and once this was completed a visit was organized with both the owner and the loaner present. When the loaner demonstrated the horse's actions, it gave a perfect repetition of the problem experienced, normally quite a rare occurrence in the field of behavioural consultancy. The owner watched with interest, and was then asked to try to lead the horse to the field to see if this made any difference in the behaviour demonstrated by the horse. Almost immediately the horse allowed the owner to lead it to the field, therefore confirming the problem appeared to originate with the loaner. All other aspects of the loan were going well, and the horse was ridden in the school and hacked out regularly with no issues. This appeared to be a case where the horse was for some reason unsure of the loaner on the ground, even when they repeated exactly the actions of the owner. In this case the origin of the problem seemed to be a mystery, and the routine of the horse was assessed until it was discovered that normally the horse would be led out first away from its stable companions as the loaner worked early in the morning. The reason why the horse would lead with the owner was not apparent, but judged to be probable familiarity with its usual caregiver and therefore be classically conditioned to be more in harmony from any instruction given by them. A programme of retraining to familiarize the horse with the loaner was devised, incorporating leading, school work, grooming and light massage sessions to increase familiarity on the ground (Fig. 4.8). The pair had no behavioural issues while riding, which made for an interesting discussion regarding the reasons behind this odd case study. After the retraining had taken place the horse was able to be led to the field by the loaner, and they also reported the horse to be calmer and more relaxed out riding than it had been before.

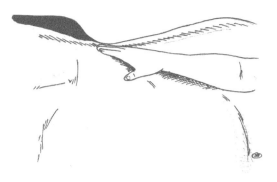

Fig. 4.8. Light massage sessions can help to reduce tension in stressed horses.

Case study 2

The ridden case study concerned a young mare who presented with the classic signs of napping: failure to progress out through the entrance of the livery yard, suddenly, with no build-up of behaviours or previous warnings. As with the previous case, every other factor was checked and the medical history of the horse was examined. The rider had asked for help from the livery owners, and various methods such as circling and then attempting to walk forwards had been trialled, along with using a crop to intensify the leg signals. The rider dismounted and was asked to discuss any recent events experienced by the horse out hacking, anything that might have caused this sudden refusal to walk forwards. Nothing was discovered, or identified, so a process of retraining was put in place for the horse, involving a return to some foundation training to try to solve the problem by reinforcing forward movement at a basic level. The training was started immediately, to gauge acceptance, with the mare having her tack left in place and two lunge lines attached to the bit rings to long-rein her instead of being ridden.

The mare began the programme of retraining, with a period of long-reining undertaken three times a week, starting around the livery yard and in the school and slowly progressing through the gates and out on to the lanes. The mare was only taken out for short distances at first, then these were increased until she was moving forwards and striding out on the walks. The rider still rode her in the school, but concentrated on exercises such as changing transitions to improve contact, length of stride and onward motion. The time came when the rider wanted to trial taking the mare outside the gates, so after a short period of long-reining in the school she mounted up and rode straight towards the entrance, keeping a clear contact and making sure the mare knew what she was asking her to do. They reached the entrance and the mare did hesitate at first, but then strode out through the gates, to the extreme pleasure of her rider. It was reported that the horse did often start to waver before the entrance was reached, but with gentle persuasion she never stopped again and the pair were able to enjoy the countryside once more.

Case study 3

The last case was another where the origin of the behaviour remained undiscovered, and it involved a large warmblood used for unaffiliated dressage that had suddenly begun to stop as soon as it approached one corner of the school. A visit was organized and the horse was observed in the school, demonstrating the behaviour as described. Once the horse napped, the owner could not get it

anywhere near this same corner and had to ride out into the school off the track to avoid the corner and then could manoeuvre the horse back on to the track (Fig. 4.9). This unusual behaviour continued whatever gait the horse moved in, and also the direction, either left or right, did not matter. The horse also appeared quite stressed, performing conflict behaviours on the approach to the corner, and also looking quite distressed much of the time. The owner could not think of anything that had caused the behaviour, or any particular event when it had started to nap as it was ridden into the corner.

After the situation was discussed, the solution to the problem seemed to lie within the process of positive reinforcement, due to the use of this in operant conditioning in reducing stress response in the horse. The solution seemed simple: a helper would stand in the offending corner with some sort of treat used as a reward that was very motivating and appetitive for the horse. The idea involved this use of operant conditioning, with a positive reinforcer (the treat) given as a reward to the horse

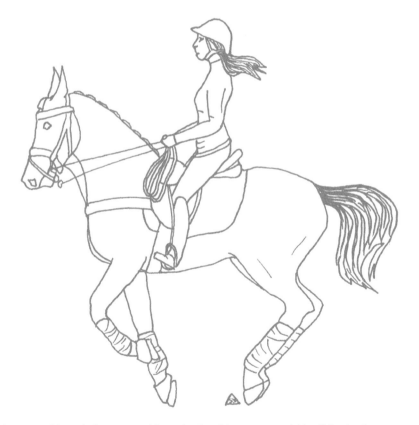

Fig. 4.9. The horse would nap in the corner of the school and jump away quickly off the track.

once they entered the area of the corner in the school. The owner decided they wanted to ride, rather than lead or long-rein due to the size of the horse, so the helper was positioned with a bag of treats and the experiment began. As the horse approached the corner for the first time, the helper moved out of the corner to give the horse a reward and shape the forward movement towards the frightening area. The owner rode the horse around, and this time the approach seemed a little less stressful and the treat accepted slightly closer to the corner. The method continued for a few more circuits and then repeated over the next couple of days until the horse could be ridden straight into the corner. The helper then moved away out of the school, and there was no change in the behaviour – the owner could still ride right into the troublesome corner in both directions and in all three gaits. This was a rather special case study, and a very satisfying one to solve with adherence to positive reinforcement that is so often overlooked as impractical in horse training due to the involvement of treat rewards.

Jogging

The behaviour of jogging is described as the swift short-striding trot commonly seen when out hacking, perhaps in combination with heading home, or in arousing conditions for the horse, for example heading to a place where it generally goes for a gallop. Horses as prey animals are intrinsically linked with locomotion, and the size of their cerebellum where movement is processed seems larger in scale than many other animals (Fig. 4.10). However, research regarding the processes of the cerebellum in the horse is limited (Scott *et al.*, 2018), so most knowledge of this part of the brain relates to other species and the

structure and function can only be interpreted along with other prey animals. This explanation certainly has some bearing on the behaviour of the horse, and particularly with locomotive behavioural problems such as jogging and bolting. When a horse speeds up in this way, it is merely motivated to get somewhere else, or to leave danger behind, and in the case of jogging it is explained as a motivational need to move faster than it is being allowed to do. Going from a walk into a trot obviously speeds up motion, and if the rider is trying to slow the horse down by pulling on the reins it may slow enough to shorten the stride of its trot but not enough to transition down to a walk. The rider is left with a rather frustrating short, choppy trot motion that the horse trials in situations where it is aroused and is one of those behaviours that will easily become classically conditioned wherever the situation repeats itself – for instance heading home.

The jogging horse is merely acting out its natural behaviour, and as such this can be a very difficult problem to solve, due to the ongoing reinforcement of gaining reward every time it is repeated. Horses performing the behaviour need to be placed in a position where jogging is not rewarded by forward movement and is slowly extinguished when the reward is not forthcoming. The difficulty with problem locomotory actions is the aspect of hard-wired behaviour: the faster the horse goes, the more it builds on its reward. The main theory in reducing these locomotory problem behaviours is to slow the horse, whatever the situation, so that the heart rate reduces naturally and arousal is diminished (Fig. 4.11). Therefore, dealing with this behavioural issue needs a patient rider, who is prepared to spend some time asking the horse to transition back to walk every time it begins to jog and not getting impatient every time it happens. This appears to work better than any other method so far experienced, and certainly seems a simpler solution than turning the horse to hack for a longer distance every time it jogs, as eventually the horse will need to head home. Other traditional methods include circling the horse when it jogs, making it come to a complete stop each time and trialling stronger and thinner bits. None of these proposed solutions really act on reducing arousal, as for example pressure from the bit if asked to stop completely will need to be strong and uncompromising, further accelerating the stress response.

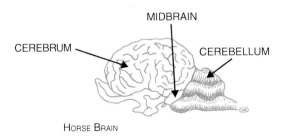

MIDBRAIN

CEREBRUM

CEREBELLUM

HORSE BRAIN

Fig. 4.10. The cerebellum in the horse is a large part of the volume of its brain.

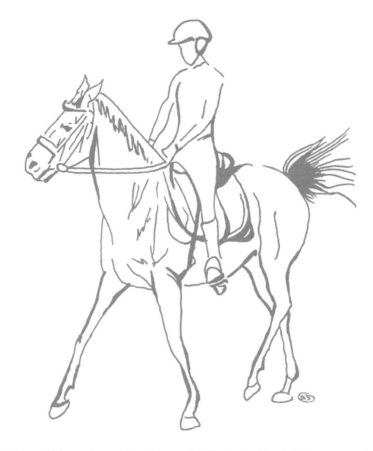

Fig. 4.11. A jogging horse ridden on the road can be very irritating to its rider, but also poses a danger as is generally not listening to any instruction.

- As jogging is linked to the flight behavioural repertoire, it is recommended to try to slow the horse to reduce its arousal, rather than resort to methods that increase it.
- Using negative reinforcement to ask the horse to slow, and then making sure the reward of pressure-release is accurate seems to lessen arousal.
- Accuracy in using negative reinforcement is paramount with this problem behaviour.

Take-home message

Use a rider who is very skilled in applying negative reinforcement and is patient in dealing with horses.

Case study

The lively cob involved in this case study belonged to a rider who loved all the exciting rides, going through the woods, the local beach and on steep tracks. This horse was therefore quite a hyperactive type and fitted well with its owner, both of them really elucidating the term 'happy hacker'. Problems with jogging only really began to develop when the owner was unable to ride for a few weeks, and someone else rode the cob out as a favour. Very soon the horse began to jog on rides, mainly once turned for home but also approaching the woods or the beach. This was mentioned to the owner once they started riding the cob again, and it soon became apparent the that the horse had not changed and performed the same behaviours as with the other person. A call-out was arranged, and the cob was observed jogging at various places along the route, becoming worse as the rider tried to stop the jogging and bring them back to walk. As the cob was observed, a procedure to retrain and attempt to extinguish the jogging became evident and the pair were followed back to the yard.

A session held with the owner explained how negative reinforcement worked, with clear pressure-release on the slightest slowing of the horse, and endeavouring to make sure they were not hanging on to the reins all the time but giving and taking with the horse's movement. A couple of schooling sessions followed, with the owner perfecting their pressure-release skills until the horse was responding quickly to a progressively lighter signal to slow their pace. It was up to the owner now to take the horse on a hack and practise what they had learnt once the horse started to jog. Results were not seen for a little while, but the owner reported the horse was beginning to stop using jogging as its hard-wired go-to behaviour when it became excited. The slowing of the horse back to a walk each time it jogged, therefore denying it the reward of faster movement, appeared to be solving the problem, and soon the horse rarely jogged as the behaviour became extinguished. The owner reported a year or so later that the cob still jogged on occasion, but they knew how to stop the problem escalating and had even taken part in some successful organized 'fun' rides.

Shying

Shying is a very common problem behaviour in horses, linked to their evolution as a prey animal, where running at the first sign of danger can ensure their safety. To the rider, or handler, this action can be very dangerous, as in the most extreme cases some horses will not consider any objects or barriers around them and can try to run straight through, causing injury to themselves or their handlers/riders. It must be considered that this is a natural behaviour for a horse, therefore it is a feature of their behavioural repertoire in which it is very difficult, if not impossible, to train them to behave otherwise. Foundation training needs to have a real emphasis on introducing the young horse to novel objects, vehicles, trailers, jumps and everything they may encounter, until they are acknowledged to be generalizing their reactions to these new encounters (Fig. 4.12). Every horse will have its own personality and it is obvious to their handlers, even very early on in foundation training, whether an animal will be one who is naturally more hyperactive, or less reactive, or perhaps quieter to handle. Indeed, when riders were asked to compare and rank the temperamental peculiarities of a group of horses, they all agreed with each other (Visser *et al.*, 2003). This would seem to suggest horsepersons are very good judges of horses, though whether this can also

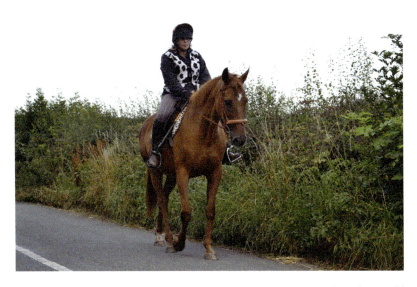

Fig. 4.12. Hacking on the roads can be dangerous due to the many novel situations that arise, so riders are encouraged to train their horses to be as unreactive as possible.

relate to their ability to select the best partnerships is relatively unknown. Accordingly, consideration of the rider is essential, and it has been reported that if a horse is of a hyperactive temperament, the relationships with individual riders can affect cooperation whereas it does not with more passive animals (Visser *et al.*, 2008).

Consequently, horses in their foundation training need to be trained carefully in their approach to novel objects, by the person most fitted for the task depending on their temperament (Fig. 4.13). Additionally, when choosing a horse for a hack, riders must make the same considerations of their own temperament and that of the horse itself. It is never a good idea to match a tense horse with a nervous rider, and when shying is taken into consideration the rider needs to be able to keep calm, work through the problem and not to panic in what can be very dangerous situations, particularly if they are on a road. If the problem involves a newly purchased horse, or an unfamiliar rider, the shying

behaviour can be amplified, as horses will have a reduced fear response if they are with a familiar handler or rider (Marsboll and Christensen, 2015). It appears then that any retraining for horses fearful of novel objects needs to be undertaken by a familiar handler, and one who knows the horse's temperament and how best to handle them.

The consideration of the act of shying is very important, and sometimes quite confusing to those handling such horses. Indeed, it is anecdotally reported there is no such thing as a 'bombproof horse', and every animal may one day meet an object that scares it, or it sees danger in something very unexpected such as a plastic bag. To those involved with horses who cannot understand how a slight movement in the hedgerow is so terrifying to a horse, yet a large vehicle provokes no reaction at all, this may be explained in evolutionary terms. That moving leaf at the side of the road may in fact hide a predator and this could well be an innate reaction to something that could prove extremely

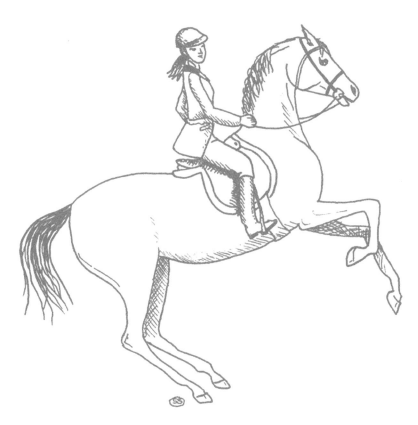

Fig. 4.13. If a horse shies when out on a hack it is important to introduce it carefully to the object – any attempt at pushing the horse or using a whip may result in a slight rearing action.

dangerous, until it is investigated and seen to be safe. As for the large vehicle, on the other hand: if the horse has not had an aversive encounter with one it may just be that – a vehicle that is big and noisy, yes, but as it has never posed a threat in the past, why would it now? These thoughts can then apply to every situation where a horse shies away at something. The horse is not stupid or silly; it is merely reacting to something that really could kill it – a possible predator hiding in the bushes.

Horses presenting with shying problems are therefore best put in a programme of retraining involving exposure to many varied novel objects, whether it is being ridden around the yard, in a school or indeed on the road with a cohort of herd companions. Once a novel object is sighted, the horse should be asked to approach it, however slowly it needs to, and allowed to back away only to turn it around again with the least amount of pressure. The horse will eventually want to interact with the object, usually by touching it with its muzzle, and this is to be encouraged. After the horse fully accepts the novelty, the training can continue until the next time the horse shies and so on. Nevertheless, problems can occur with the approach to novel objects where the horse is extremely agitated, or stressed by the circumstance, and if this occurs in a dangerous area such as a road then safety must be considered. It is reported that horses have far less reaction to novel objects when they are led in hand, rather than ridden (von Borstel *et al.*, 2011), so sometimes it is good to dismount and lead the horse up to and eventually past the offending item. It is not recommended to escalate the situation by the horse being hit with a whip, or shouted at, making it even more fearful and therefore actually punishing it for what is only natural behaviour. Worsening the situation in this way will harm the horse's ability to learn, its reaction in the future and its relationship with the rider, so horsepersons must be responsible and act calmly and defuse the incident.

Key points

- Shying is a natural evolved behaviour for horses, so they should never be punished for it.
- Horses and riders must be matched for temperament as far as is possible, and this needs to be taken into consideration if a horse is known for shying.
- Plenty of positive reinforcement and patience reduces the horse's stress, so is very pertinent in

a situation where by bolting off or bucking the horse could put itself or people in danger.
- It is not a failure if the rider needs to dismount and lead the horse past a frightening object – this enables stress levels to reduce and presents the horse with an opportunity to accept and learn from the experience.

Take-home message

Horses have evolved to run from dangerous circumstances. It is the rider's or handler's responsibility to reduce the reaction to these fears and retrain where necessary, in methods that decrease stress and enable learning to occur.

Case study 1

A very handsome Welsh Cob was the subject of a case study concerning shying, where the ultimate resolution was a little different to what might be assumed. The owner was really struggling with the pony, and it was already becoming more fearful as each ride took place – shying at objects it had never reacted to before, and intensifying those reactions. The pony mysteriously seemed to react completely differently in its field, where it was ridden by another rider and jumped over various structures, galloping around with no shying evident even when dogs were walked along the nearby footpath. The behavioural consultant came to visit the pony, and to watch it in the field and on a hack. It was apparent very quickly that there was quite a difference between the two riders, concerning confidence and riding ability. The rider who took the pony around the field was fearless, and it seemed the pony reacted in some way to this, even though it did shy at some things where the rider was confident enough to let the pony slow, and approach the object, before riding on. When the owner was observed hacking the pony out, it could have been a different animal, reactive, tense and demonstrating quite a few conflict behaviours.

Unfortunately, this case could only be solved by honesty – the owner was asked carefully about their confidence and ability, and it was discussed that the reason the horse did not appear to shy in the field was due to the reassurances of the other rider. This was proved by the other rider taking the cob on a hack, where it experienced the same objects it would shy at with the owner, but provoking no reaction when ridden by the other rider. Solutions were discussed to include a retraining programme going back to foundation training for the cob; however, it was explained this was unlikely to change its temperament, only perhaps allowing it to handle new experiences a little more calmly. The only other solution was for the owner to gain additional proficiency with other horses and have some riding lessons to improve their confidence, so they could then be more able to ride the horse and handle its shying episodes.

Case study 2

The second case study involved a warmblood, large enough to cause problems for its owner when it shied in the dressage arena. There was a set pattern for this horse. At home it hardly ever shied without there being a sufficient reason; it just appeared to happen when it was performing at shows and there were plant pots or other objects placed around the dressage boards. The owner had been very proactive with the horse, and had placed her own plants and items in her own school, where the horse continually ignored them and did not react at all. The next show the horse attended did involve some plant arrangements at the side of the arena, and a full observation of the animal took place to ascertain some sort of reason for its behaviour. As the observation took place, the horse did indeed shy at the plants, and continued to do so a few more times as it was ridden in the test. The movements were not huge, nor dangerous, just enough for the rider to be marked down in their test. The key to the reactions appeared to be the state of arousal of the horse: in a normal ridden exercise at home it would not react but as soon as it was put under different stresses this was enough to raise its awareness and cause the problem to arise.

The solution was perhaps easy, but needed some additional thinking in how to solve it. The owner had tried with pots at home, but not the increased amount of people watching, so this had to be trialled to establish if the presence of a crowd was enough to heighten the horse's arousal state. It could also be other factors, such as the travel time in the trailer, but the first idea was tried before this was considered. The plan was to put in place a small crowd at the horse's home arena involving other livery owners, providing an audience to see if this raised the horse's stress levels enough for it to start shying. The arena was marked out with dressage boards, and plant pots and the people were placed in position. The owner rode the horse into the marked-out area and, as hoped, the horse shied at the plants, so under instruction they kept riding it around, approaching the pots and letting it sniff them with its muzzle. They approached different plants and noted the reactions as they began to lessen. Then the horse was ridden out of the arena, only to be brought back in once the pots had been moved around. This exercise was repeated a couple of times a week, with some different objects, up to the date of their next show, and this was attended by the behaviourist to determine any difference in behaviour. After the test, the horse did get a much-improved result than it would normally have received, and even though it still did look at some of the pots there was not enough reaction to score the horse down too badly. The owner continued to ride the horse at home sometimes with the addition of a small crowd, and over time there were improvements with all its scores (Fig. 4.14).

Bucking

The action of bucking is related to evolutionary adaptation and it is thought to be a mechanism for a prey animal to try to dislodge a predator from their back (Fig. 4.15). Bucking is sometimes seen by riders as not a worrisome problem, if it happens when the horse tends to buck at the start of a canter, or when they are in an aroused state. When owners were questioned, bucking was denoted as a problem in only 1.9% of horses (Bachmann and Stauffacher, 2002), further corroborating the anecdotal evidence that bucking is not seen as particularly problematic by most riders. If riders are experienced, and their horses do buck occasionally, this may not be seen as a problem at all, and those horses handled by professional riders do anyway appear to have a lesser frequency of bucking (Kydd et al., 2017). This may be due to a more correct approach to the use of negative reinforcement, so a professional rider might understand that the horse needs rewarding with pressure-release once it has performed the wanted action, such as slowing down. Interestingly there is also some research linking poor performance to bucking (Buckley et al., 2004), so this factor may indeed persuade professionals to investigate it. Nevertheless, injuries to riders when mounted are more likely to involve medical care at a hospital rather than those while the person is engaged in groundwork, so it is a

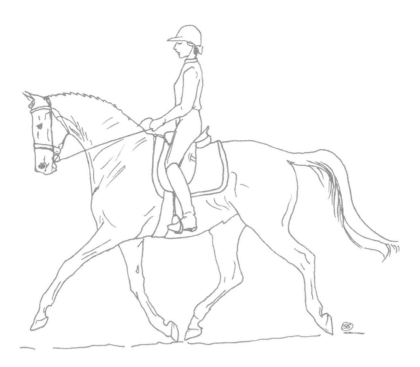

Fig. 4.14. After training with the pot plants and other objects, the horse's dressage test results improved significantly.

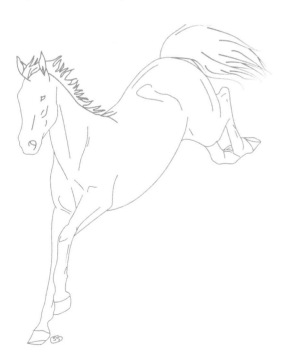

Fig. 4.15. A buck from a horse with its head raised is much easier to sit and is generally thought to be an expression of excitement rather than pain.

problem that needs some attention due to safety issues if it occurs frequently (Acton *et al.*, 2019).

Bucking has been related to sacro-iliac joint pain (Barstow and Dyson, 2015) amongst other issues, including incorrect saddle fitting and dental complications. There is always the possibility of bucking being directly related to a pain issue, so it is always advised that a thorough veterinary examination is carried out, and also saddle fitting to determine that none of these factors are causing any issues. Once the horse has been examined fully, if it is still bucking it is prudent to investigate tack and if any artificial aids are being used, and an observation carried out by a qualified professional may identify the cause. If there appears to be no underlying cause the horse needs to be assessed very carefully, as bucking takes many different forms such as fly-bucking, where the head is raised, or a full buck where the head is lowered and the rider, if not secure, may end up going over the horse's head (Fig. 4.16). A secure and confident rider is a must with bucking problems, as the horse will possibly benefit from a return to foundation training to try to reduce stress. Environmental conditions must also be considered in any retraining plan, as horses have been reported to buck more if

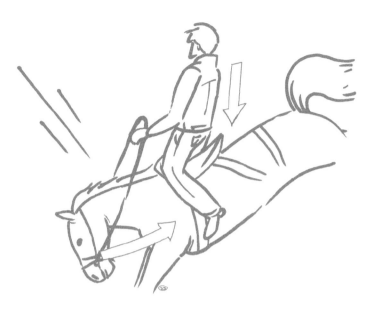

Fig. 4.16. A buck where the head is lowered is much more difficult to sit for a rider, and in an emergency the horse should be pulled upwards and the rider should sit down in the saddle.

they are confined in their stable even for a single day (Jung *et* al., 2019). Consequently, bucking can be associated with lack of turnout, so a retraining programme may need an element of increased paddock-time included. Nutrition must also be considered, where excess energy may involve an increase in the behaviour due to higher arousal.

Each circumstance must therefore be individually tailored to the horse in question, with a consideration for the environment in which the horse will be working. Stress and frustration appear to be the underlying factors causing behaviour-related bucking, so a foundation retraining programme may include the use of negative reinforcement. The horse could be returned to groundwork and correct leading before possibly using long-reining, and only then progressing to ridden work, enabling the animal to relearn in a more relaxed situation. Any pressure-release needs to be very accurate to avoid confusion, and the prevalence of conflict behaviour should be noted carefully as this may well indicate to an observer when the horse is experiencing high levels of frustration and needs to return to a previous step in their retraining. Taken slowly and with consideration, horses with bucking issues can return to work after a period of retraining. This may illustrate an extinction of the behaviour where the horse has not been pressurized into the unknown circumstance that caused the initial bucking, so has no reason to display it again.

Key points

- As bucking is highly correlated with pain, horses displaying this problem behaviour need to be fully investigated.
- Do not forget to examine the likelihood of any husbandry factors that may be contributing to the behaviour.
- Usually a programme of retraining involving a return to foundation work will reduce stress for the horse concerned, and though it may take time the problem behaviour may be extinguished once the motivation to perform it is removed.

Take-home message

Bucking must be investigated fully to ensure that pain or discomfort is not the underlying issue.

Case study 1

A pony successful in local shows began to buck, and at first displayed small bucks easily coped with by its young rider. However, over a period of time these apparently began to develop into dangerous unseating behaviours and a thorough examination by the vet, saddler and equine dentist took place before the behaviourist was called out. An observation of the pony raised a few questions, and it became clear the animal was only 5 years old, and had already competed in classes throughout its 5th year. The tendency to buck appeared when the pony was experiencing higher levels of arousal, such as jumping, or cantering in a field, and always at shows. The young rider was a little 'handy' with the whip when the pony displayed conflict behaviours, and on observation this only increased the likelihood of it bucking.

Several issues had to be faced. The young rider needed to stop using the whip the way they were, as a punishment when the pony bucked, and needed some refinement to their natural aids to enable them to signal the pony more accurately. Their use of negative reinforcement did not engage any pressure-release, so the pony was constantly learning that the incessant kicking and pulling on the reins did not relent and involved no reward for it to respond to. The real danger of the development of some sort of psychological condition was explained to the owner. Also, after some discussion it was suggested that the pony had perhaps not had time to adapt in its youthful career, and would benefit from a short period of respite before retraining took place.

The pony enjoyed a short break, still being handled daily for grooming and health care, but no attempt made to ride or work with it beyond leading to and from the paddock. When this was carried out, the young rider learned the basics of pressure-release, and appreciated how quickly the pony responded to the training. Once the break was over, the pony began to retrain with a foundation programme, starting with some long-reining and progressing to slow walking around the school and on short hacks. Trotting was included in the programme, and eventually cantering, all with no pressure and understanding shown when the pony appeared to need a retrograde move before again proceeding. Eventually the pony was ready to return to some local shows, again reducing pressure and stress where possible, and the young rider was now able to forget about the bucking period and enjoy riding once again.

Case study 2

The second case study is a very short one, and involved a large cob at a riding school who began to buck for no apparent reason. All the checks where done, different riders experimented with, but to no avail. The cob still bucked, regularly throwing off riders, and eventually causing injury. The horse had to leave the riding school, and a home was found for it firstly as a companion pony. Luckily this did happen, and the horse went to a new home where it was given a month off work completely, with plenty of turn-out and companionship. The horse was checked again, and no problems found, so the new owner began to take it out for slow hacks. Intriguingly, the change of environment and use of the cob possibly afforded it with no motivation to repeat its previous behaviour, and certainly it did not buck again. A change of environment is not always possible, but must be considered in situations where conflict behaviours seem to be out of character and unusual for the individual concerned.

Bolting

The origin of bolting is quite clear: in its evolution from the forests to the plains the small mammal that became the horse needed to adapt to its changing environment and learn to run and not hide. These adaptations of the horse were extremely successful in their development as a prey animal able to run almost from birth. The horse evolved to possess a smaller digestive system than other grazers to limit weight, one hardened toe to speed up pace, no clavicles and a fixed spine to allow a longer stride and the ability to produce at least a third more blood cells instantaneously from its spleen to increase oxygen supply. All these factors led to the modern-day athlete that is the horse, and around 5000 years of domestication is probably not enough to change its basic maintenance behaviours. Therefore, the horse's innate behaviour in circumstances where danger (or perceived danger) suddenly appears is to run. The foundation training a horse receives needs to address this natural behaviour of bolting and condition the horse not to return to its use when it identifies a possible threatening situation. The use of learning theory in a foundation training programme will work to reduce the stress shown around novel objects, using desensitization to introduce new circumstances, encompass the correct use of negative and positive reinforcement and avoid punishment at every level. When asking the horse to work faster, it should never be encouraged to speed up without the ability to slow it down, and this may therefore exclude the use of lungeing if the horse is inclined to increase its pace out of control.

As discussed, there is evidence to suggest that lungeing and the practice of round-pen may hardwire a horse to perform the behaviour of bolting, as when it speeds up in these conditions it is not generally asked to slow down and in the case of round-pen it is encouraged to go faster. A horse that is fresh may be lunged before work to expend its energy, possibly detrimental to what the handler is essentially trying to achieve. Anecdotally, horses are also ridden at fast paces to reduce their excitement or lessen their energy, but if this is hardwiring the horse to revert to this behaviour it is perhaps not recommended. However, in a survey where owners reported problem behaviours, only 3% stated that their horses had bolted in the week before the data collection (Hockenhull and Creighton, 2013), suggesting it may not be as common as is thought. Consequently, using any methods that encourage a horse to run faster may produce an animal more inclined to bolt in its daily work, and it is perhaps better advised for foundation training not to include any of these methods.

The horse that has begun to bolt as a go-to behaviour will need careful treatment, and the use of experienced riders able to cope in these circumstances. There must be a veterinary examination, and an inspection must include the saddle and bridle and in particular the type of bit or bitless bridle in use. These horses often benefit from reducing the severity of the bridle/bit in use, in contrast to what might be expected. The use of increasingly severe bits will escalate quite quickly, and the horse may start to develop other conflict behaviours along with the bolting due to pain or discomfort. This indicates that the horse in question needs to return to a retraining programme with some elements of foundation training involved. Leading training using negative reinforcement will begin to have effects on the horse once it is ridden, and certainly calm and relaxed schooling where attention is paid to downward transitions will help to restore a light contact and control to the rider. The presence of well-trained herd companions to accompany the horse on leisurely hacks will also help at first, so if a bolting behaviour does occur the horse may well be encouraged not to run too far and to slow down. If any such behaviour does happen it is imperative that everything is tried to slow the horse down to reduce the reward of the horse getting away from the frightening object. Slowing the horse in the state of bolting removes reinforcement of the behaviour and will eventually act to extinguish it. However, as bolting is such an innate action for a horse to perform, it may take patience and time to remove it completely.

Key points

- Bolting is an innate behaviour difficult to extinguish once it becomes the go-to for the horse.
- There is perhaps no place in foundation training for methods that use a process of chasing, as this may reinforce bolting behaviour.
- If a horse bolts, every effort must be made to stop it as soon as possible.

Take-home message

There is a need for further research into the effects of training methods that include chasing as part of their techniques.

Case study

The mare involved in this case study had a slightly different problem than most bolting horses, and many techniques were trialled to attempt to solve it. The horse was an older ex-hunt master's horse, whose current owner was not particularly worried that the horse ran away with them, as they tended to stop once they reached the end of familiar gallops. However, the problem lay with those who accompanied them on rides, and these included an ex-racehorse with a flighty temperament and a younger person's pony; these people thought the problem needed to be solved for safety reasons as the owner of the mare was quite elderly. Once the mare was observed on a gallop close to the yard where the horses were kept, it was clear it was a very habituated behaviour – there appeared to be no fearful responses, just the stimulus of reaching the usual gallop track and setting off in what looked like a completely uncontrollable speed. It was apparent the situation had been happening for a long time, and the success of solving it considered as quite low.

In the past the owner had been advised to try methods such as riding on draw reins to pull the horse's head down in a more controllable position, or try stronger bits, or circle it around and maybe as a last resort running the horse into a hedge. None of these methods had worked (and luckily they had not tried the last suggestion), so the situation remained unsolved. The horse did not appear to be worried where its herd companions were and would bolt off into gallop whether on its own or with others. The riding tracks and bridle paths available to the yard were extensive and very varied, including one through a wood, which was the only place where the mare did not break into a gallop, possibly due to obstacles such as tree stumps and the need to stop and start again around a few trees. The possibility of using this track only for fast work to retrain the horse had been tried in the past, but as soon as they had returned to the flat gallops the animal reverted to its customary behaviour.

No simple solution presented itself, and any retraining suggestions seemed to need a change of rider to someone a little more experienced with whom the horse was not used to running away (Fig. 4.17). This seemed to be the key, and feasibly the answer to solving the bolting dilemma with this particular horse. Permission was sought from the owner, and a local trainer who used to ride racehorses and who was also friendly with the owner offered to help. They were provided with a quick introduction to how negative reinforcement works and asked to make sure any reduction in pace was rewarded straight away. Routes were devised on the extensive bridle path network, so the horse and rider entered a known gallop very close to its ending, not permitting the horse to be able to speed up very much before it had to slow. After the parameters were in place, the pair hacked to the first

location where the turn into the gallop was along a hedge, and the observation took place. The new rider was far more capable of holding the horse, and made sure the horse was rewarded for any response to aids for slowing down. After this small success, the pair hacked out a few times every week, with the owner of the horse taking the advantage to ride another, safer animal to learn how to use negative reinforcement correctly and experience what it felt like for a horse to respond to signals.

Another visit was arranged for a month's time and the pair were observed on the gallop tracks, where it was apparent that the horse had stopped galloping off at every opportunity it had and would, while not quietly cantering to the end of a track, certainly be far more controllable. However, since this period of retraining had taken place, the owner had become very settled with the other horse and was now not sure they wanted to return to riding the mare. So although the problem was partially solved, the mare went to be a hack with the trainer, and the original owner arranged to ride the safer horse on a regular basis. Not every case study ends up with complete resolution, but in this circumstance the result for all parties appeared to work well.

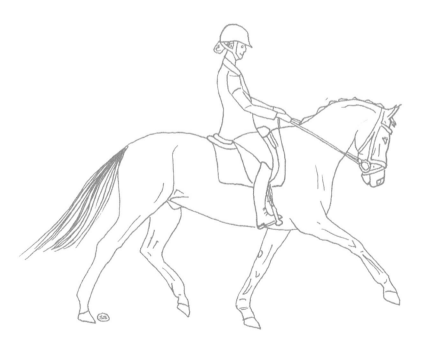

Fig. 4.17. With any behavioural problem, it is possible that the rider may be over-horsed and this cannot be overlooked.

Rearing

The prevalence of rearing has been reported by owners at 7% in leisure horses (Hockenhull and Creighton, 2013), seemingly quite a small amount but still representing a large number of horses with a behaviour problem that is dangerous and can potentially be fatal to either party (Fig. 4.18). The origin of rearing as a behaviour is probably a combination of striking out at a predator when cornered and also in the stallion's fighting repertoire. It must be noted, however, that actual fighting between rival stallions is rare, and usually warnings are enough before any injury is caused. Rearing can therefore be described as a behaviour occurring when the horse is feeling trapped and cannot flee, or in some circumstances if it is being made to do something that for whatever reason is very aversive to it. An example of the first may be a horse having a medical procedure that is cornered in a stable – the animal may rear up and even strike out to stop it happening. For the second, it could be a horse being whipped to force it over a jump that for some reason it sees as dangerous – and the rider or handler needs to remember that what seems threatening to a horse may appear perfectly reasonable to a human. The real issue with rearing in any of these circumstances is that the behaviour often quickly becomes hard-wired, and then a habitual reaction to any situation the horse feels uncomfortable in, even if it is something the animal would usually not react to (Fig. 4.19).

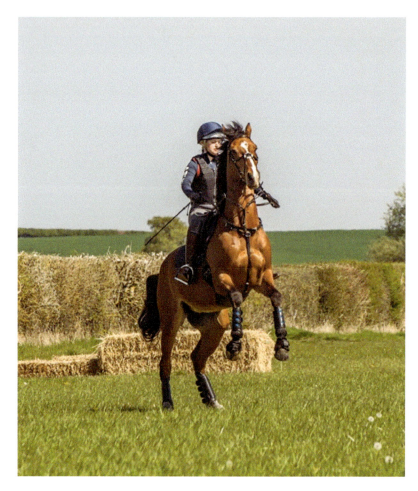

Fig. 4.18. A horse rearing on a cross-country training day – circumstances lend themselves to a rise in the arousal of the animal.

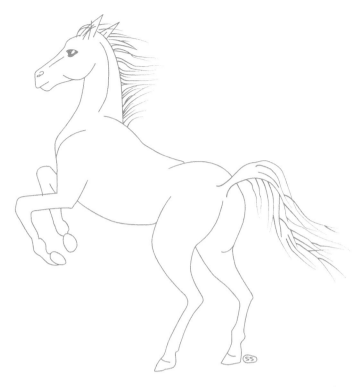

Fig. 4.19. Rearing can quickly become a 'go-to' behaviour and trialled whenever the horse is put under stress.

As a ridden problem, rearing is extremely difficult to extinguish – it develops quickly as a go-to behaviour for the horse, and many riders and handlers would naturally report it as one of the most difficult to stop a horse performing. For this reason, many techniques have been suggested for 'rearers' – horses confirmed as those who trial the behaviour whenever they are put under a certain degree of pressure. These are as varied as cracking an egg over the horse's head to give it the impression they are wounded and need to stop the action, to actually pulling the horse over backwards, jumping off and letting it crash to the floor to 'teach it a lesson'. Perhaps the reason for some of these methods, and certainly the drastic ones, is owing to the danger of the problem, and the risk it has for riders and handlers alike.

In common with many behavioural problems, rearing may be associated with pain or discomfort, so certainly with a horse that has never reared before, and suddenly starts doing so, a full veterinary examination is advised. There are incidences where brain tumours have been found in confirmed rearers once an autopsy has been performed, and

some have reported other painful causes such as tooth abscesses and even impinged spinal processes ('kissing' spine syndrome). Once any medical issues have been rejected, it is very helpful to know what, if anything, started the behaviour, when it was first experienced and all the circumstances surrounding it. Horses will generally, though not always, pivot on one leg when they are rearing, and if this is the case the retraining will to some extent concentrate on making it demanding for the horse to repeat by only using the rein on the opposite side – pulled down and laterally – to throw the weight of the horse on to the other leg. Sometimes this is enough to stop the horse rearing altogether, especially if administered early in the behaviour's progress by a confident rider possessing a good seat. The rider needs to maintain good balance, and throw themselves forward when the rear takes place to avoid overbalancing the horse, as the action of falling backwards on to the ground can injure the horse and in the worst-case scenario cause them to land on the rider.

If the horse is already using rearing as its go-to behaviour when aversive circumstances are experienced, there is a real need to revert to foundation training and return to work that the horse finds comfortable to accomplish. For example, if the horse only rears during ridden work, it may be sensible to return to groundwork for a period of time to relax the horse and not put it under any pressure. If the horse only rears during competitions, it may need some work at home and then a gradual return. The aim with this work is to eliminate the stressful circumstances the horse is asked to perform in and concentrate on those the horse does well and seems to be relaxed with. This can over time act to extinguish the rearing behaviour, and then when the horse has its work systematically increased to the levels it can cope with, the behaviour does not make a reappearance. With a horse rearing in hand, the same technique could be followed, but it is much more difficult if the horse is rearing just in walk as there is no real regression to previous schooling before leading. In these cases, and one is explained below, the use of positive reinforcement and/or counter-conditioning is suggested, as both can be administered easily from the ground. Positive reinforcement with a rearer in hand must be easy for the handler to accomplish, with the reward process very appetitive to the horse as an individual. It is essential that the handler wears a hard hat and protective boots and gloves when retraining in this circumstance.

Key points

- If rearing starts suddenly, it is always advisable to have a full health check.
- Solutions to rearing problems are easier if the origin of the behaviour can be determined and then the affecting stimuli removed, such as over-facing at a jump or pushing a young horse too hard.
- There are different methods to deal with those horses that rear when ridden, and those rearing in hand.
- It is imperative that PPE is worn and that a confident rider is used for retraining of rearing.

Take-home message

Rearing can very easily become a go-to behaviour for a horse, and it may then trial it in unpredictable circumstances when it feels under pressure or stressed.

Case study 1

The first horse presenting with a rearing problem was a newly purchased showjumper, with no history of rearing or any other behavioural problems. It settled quite well in its new home, and was schooling calmly and carefully over poles and just beginning grid work. The horse was hacking out with its new owner, and coming into the winter they were concentrating on building the foundation for entering the new jumping season in the spring. The horse was hunted in Ireland, and the owner decided to give it something different to think about over the winter and improve the care it took over jumps and let a trusted friend take it to their local hunt. This was the trigger for the rearing to start – at first the horse appeared to thoroughly enjoy the day, jumping everything and remaining controllable for the rider. However, when the horse began to tire, and possibly should have been taken home, the rider asked it to jump a ditch and it refused. Not wanting the horse to 'learn' to stop, the rider tried to force it over and the horse went up. Luckily the rider was confident enough not to panic and brought the horse back home.

The owner gave the horse a couple of days' rest, then it was ridden again in the school and the horse went well over some ground poles and schooled well. However, when the owner tried the horse over a jump, it refused and reared again. The owner sensibly went back to the pole work and concentrated on working over those slowly to end the session rather than try a jump again. After chatting to the rider who took the horse hunting, the start of the behaviour was easily discovered, and a call-out was made to a behaviourist. As the origin of the setback was very straightforward, a programme of retraining included lots of upward transitions in the school, concentrating on asking the horse to move forward and on to the bridle. Poles were left out of the retraining for a couple of weeks, so no connection to jumping was associated to the ridden work for the horse. Once ground poles were included again, the horse was working forward very well and possibly better than before. The owner was asked to slowly reintroduce the poles and keep the speed over them but not to over-face the horse by asking it to go over too many at one time. Training continued until a small cross pole raised after three ground poles was put in place, and the horse jumped over it without any concern.

Progress was slowly controlled, but the horse never reared again, and the owner was always careful not to ask them to jump if they felt the animal was tiring or was just not ready to attempt a higher or wider jump. When the horse began competing it was taken in small classes and built up very slowly over the season until they were at the height the horse was jumping without problems before (Fig. 4.20). This case was certainly a great success, and it is thought that the reasons the horse was able to make a full recovery were the quick reactions of the rider who took the horse hunting, and the owner in not trying to pursue the problem.

Case study 2

The second case concerned an ex-racehorse that started to rear out of sheer excitement when being brought in from the field to its stable. It started in the autumn, when the grass was losing its nutritional value, and the hay and feed waiting in its stable must have proved very tempting. The horse was easy to catch, and would stand while waiting for its headcollar to be put on and the electric fence taken off its hook, but as soon as the horse started to be led it pulled strongly, reciprocated by the livery owner who then pulled it sharply back, only for the horse to go straight up in the air. This proved to be a considerable problem for the owner, as the horse had part-livery due to work commitments, and the livery owner was understandably not

happy about handling such a horse. The problem continued, with the owner having to bring the horse in later when it was dark, and this obviously corroborated the situation and made it much worse. The owner tried leading in a bridle, and then was advised to try a Chifney bit, which stopped the horse rearing, but it was so stressed that the owner decided a different solution was needed.

A visit was made when the horse was being brought in, and notes made about the distance from the field to the stable, the severity of the behaviour and the tension the horse was evidently experiencing. Solutions were discussed to find an answer to the problem, so the owner did not have to resort to using the Chifney bit as they felt the stress complicated the whole relationship and was not helping the horse at all. One solution examined the appeal of the stable environment, and the plan of removing the hay and feed until the horse was stood in the stable for a period of time was discussed, but the motivation to come in was clearly very robust and a stronger solution needed.

Leading and groundwork retraining were important to consider in this case, but as demonstrated

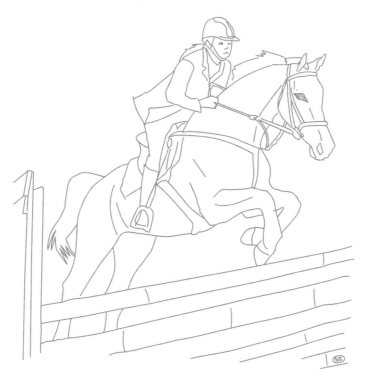

Fig. 4.20. Eventually the horse accepted jumping as part of its natural repertoire and demonstrated some success at shows.

by the owner the horse was extremely well trained and had no issues with manageability when displayed to the behaviourist. The horse would even happily stand in the school with the lead rope over its neck for the owner but would not repeat this behaviour when the motivation for it to come in was so high. Another solution presented itself, that of positive reinforcement as the horse was very motivated around food and particularly carrots, and a method of bringing the animal in with the use of this technique was trialled the next evening.

The owner made sure they had a pocket full of sliced carrots, and, once the horse was caught, immediately gave it a carrot when it stood still for the fence to be unhooked. The horse's attention came back to the owner a little, and as they moved the first couple of paces the owner asked the horse to stop and fed them another carrot. Every couple of paces the horse was asked to stand still, and on performing this behaviour it was reinforced with the obligatory reward. The horse did try to rear, but the owner stood still and gave the horse another carrot when it stood after rearing. Eventually the pair progressed down the track between the fields and through the entrance into the barn, all with only two rearing episodes and the horse a little less stressed. This method was repeated every evening, and in the morning going out to the field, so the horse really began to associate the track and its walk up and down with stopping for a reward. As the pair progressed, and rearing seemed extinguished, the owner was advised to reduce the stopping periods and walk further along the track each time with fewer reward pauses. Soon the horse could walk down the track, albeit quite fast but under control, and receive its reward at the barn entrance.

This case was noteworthy as the behaviour did not appear to be repeated in any other situation, and the groundwork with which the horse was so well trained did not readily transfer once it was very stressed. Later, it was discovered from an earlier owner that the animal was known for rearing, although it had only happened in this instance with the current owner and never when ridden. This came as quite a surprise to the owner but does further illustrate that different environments and situations affect horses significantly and in many different ways (Fig. 4.21).

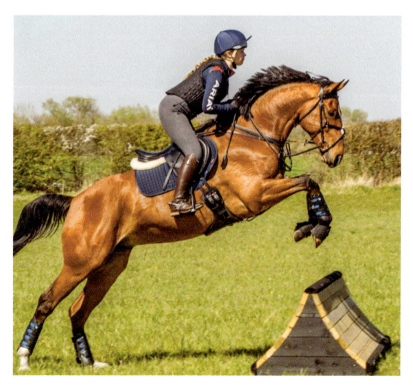

Fig. 4.21. The same horse at cross-country training showing a very good jump – its rearing episodes do not affect its performance but do add to the level of danger for the rider.

Hacking on the roads

Possibly a majority of leisure horses in the UK are ridden on the road system at some point in their lives, and many are owned specifically for this purpose. However, roads are extremely dangerous places for horses, and it may be advisable for owners not to venture on to them, but most have no choice when hacking out and indeed may have to use them to reach bridle paths and other tracks. Owing to this, horses are classed as 'vulnerable road users' and unfortunately are victims of accidents and experience near-miss incidents quite frequently (Chapman and Musselwhite, 2011). It was reported amongst Australian riders that 52% had experienced either accidents or near-misses in a period of 12 months (Thompson and Matthews, 2015). This correlates with a survey completed in the UK, where 63% of riders reported near-misses across the same period of time (Scofield *et al.*, 2013). From the end of 2010 until early 2019, according to the British Horse Society (BHS), 3737 riders reported occurrences on the road, including 43 rider deaths, 1085 injured, and 315 horses killed coupled with 945 injured (BHS, 2019). Despite these shocking figures, UK legislation has changed little to protect horse-and-rider combinations using the road network, and there also exists very little research exploring methods to keep horses and riders safer (Chapman and Musselwhite, 2011). Consequently, it is very important for riders to try any practices to keep themselves as safe as possible, while further research is carried out to look at possible education of vehicle drivers using the same road networks (Fig. 4.22).

Safety equipment

There is a plethora of available safety equipment for both horse and rider, but very little evidence to prove that any of it works to alert drivers and protect horses and riders on the road. There is evidence that wearing lights on the helmet of the rider does reduce the number of near-misses (Scofield *et al.*, 2013), as does riding coloured (piebald and skewbald) horses

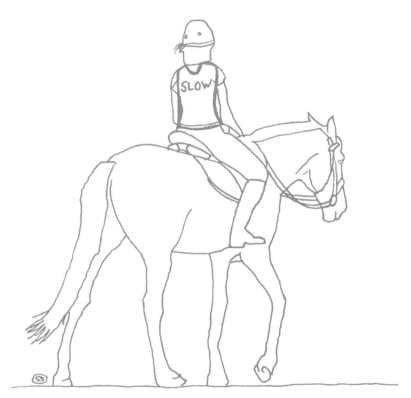

Fig. 4.22. Hacking on the roads should be a pleasure, not fraught with danger every time horse-and-rider combinations venture on to them.

(Scofield *et al.*, 2014). The finding regarding coloured horses led the author to explore other methods of conspicuity, or the characteristics of humans to see objects more clearly, and a black-and-white-tabard worn by a rider in tests showed a significant reduction in vehicle proximity to the combination (Scofield *et al.*, 2019) (Fig. 4.23). Proximity is a very important factor, as this indicates how close the vehicles pass to the horse-and-rider combination. If the horse exhibits any behaviour that would put the pair in trouble, the further the vehicle passes away from them the safer the situation. Consequently, the wearing of any conspicuity equipment is recommended, but more research is needed to ascertain what is most effective

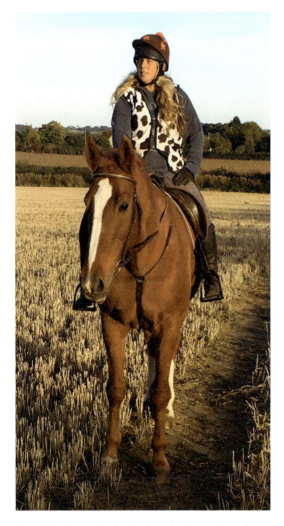

Fig. 4.23. Example of a black-and-white patterned tabard as used by the author in testing.

across different weather conditions. For example, the colour of fluorescent yellow appears to be less visible when the sun is shining (Scofield *et al.*, 2019), and naturally horse riders tend to hack on the roads more in sunny weather conditions (Scofield *et al.*, 2014).

Problems that might occur and how to avoid them

Foundation training must include a lengthy and safe introduction to the roads, all types of vehicle, and in different weather conditions. It is not safe just to train a horse when it is clement weather and forget that, in rainy weather, puddles will form and vehicles splashing through them can really spook horses. Long-reining may certainly provide a sound introduction for the young horse and having herd companions who are habituated to roads and traffic will also help. Sandwiching the young horse between two older cohorts will provide a good start, and then the horse can be moved to the front and to the back to gain experience in all positions on a ride. Long-reining the horse on its own will also help in the transition to hacking out without herd companions. Always make sure that the riders are confident and that a headcollar and lead rope are carried. When hacking out alone it is wise to let others know the route the rider is taking in case of any problems. Even if they are carrying a mobile phone, the rider may get injured and be unable to make a call.

Problem behaviours are all potentially dangerous when experienced on the roads, but bolting is possibly the most hazardous for horse-and-rider combinations, and being frightened by a vehicle may lead the horse to bolt into the path of others or the rider might lose their seat. Spooking is common, but the rider must judge when to act to improve their horse's reaction, or to accept that any horse has the capability to spook and the rider always needs be aware of a developing situation. Jogging is not so dangerous, but has consequences for horse health, fitness and the ability of the rider to hack with other combinations. Napping can delay a hack completely, so advice must be taken if this occurs. Consequently, these behaviours must be taken seriously when riders experience them, to improve the safety for both rider and horse. If the predictability of the horse by the rider can be enhanced, the whole ridden experience can be safer (Thompson *et al.*, 2015), and the use of learning theory to solve behaviour problems will make for a safer and more enjoyable hacking companion.

Conclusion

Many behavioural problems have been explored through various sections, from those experienced on the ground to ridden behaviours that impact on the enjoyment of riders and their relationships with the horses they ride. Ultimately the relationship between horse and human, whether it is a professional pairing or as a happy hacker, needs to be as safe as possible and the solving of behaviour problems in all instances can help to reinforce these very special partnerships (Figs 4.24 and 4.25).

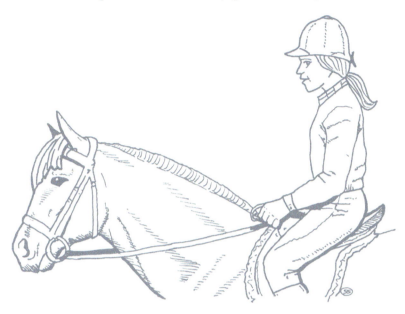

Fig. 4.24. Riding is a relationship between horse and human that should be a pleasurable experience for both parties.

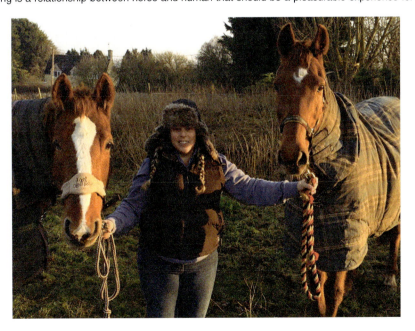

Fig. 4.25. The author.

References

Acton, A.S., Gaw, C.E., Chounthirath, T. and Smith, G.A. (2019) Nonfatal horse-related injuries treated in emergency departments in the United States, 1990–2017. *American Journal of Emergency Medicine* [in press].

Bachmann, I. and Stauffacher, M. (2002) Prevalence of behavioural disorders in the Swiss horse population. *Schweizer Archiv fur Tierheilkunde* 144(7), 356–368.

Barstow, A. and Dyson, S. (2015) Clinical features and diagnosis of sacroiliac joint region pain in 296 horses 2004–2014. *Equine Veterinary Education* 27(12), 637–647.

BHS (British Horse Society) (2019) Nearly two horses killed each week on UK roads, shocking new statistics reveal. Available at: https://www.bhs.org.uk/our-charity/press-centre/news/2019/march/dead-slow-2019 (accessed 25 April 2019).

Bowker, R.M. (2003a) Contrasting structural morphologies of 'good' and 'bad' footed horses. In: *Proceedings of the 49th Annual Convention of the American Association of Equine Practitioners*, New Orleans, Louisiana, 21–25 November 2003, pp. 186–209.

Bowker, R.M. (2003b) The growth and adaptive capabilities of the hoof wall and sole: functional changes in response to stress. In: *Proceedings of the 49th Annual Convention of the American Association of Equine Practitioners*, New Orleans, Louisiana, 21–25 November 2003, pp. 146–168.

Brunsting, J., Dumoulin, M., Oosterlinck, M., Haspeslagh, M., Lefere, L. and Pille, F. (2019) Can the hoof be shod without limiting the heel movement? A comparative study between barefoot, shoeing with conventional shoes and a split-toe shoe. *Veterinary Journal* 246, 7–11.

Buckley, P., Dunn, T. and More, S.J. (2004) Owners' perceptions of the health and performance of Pony Club horses in Australia. *Preventive Veterinary Medicine* 63(1-2), 121–133.

Chapman, C. and Musselwhite, C.B.A. (2011) Equine road user safety: public attitudes, understandings and beliefs from a qualitative study in the United Kingdom. *Accident Analysis and Prevention* 43(6), 2173–2181.

Clayton, H.M., Gray, S., Kaiser, L.J. and Bowker, R.M. (2011) Effects of barefoot trimming on hoof morphology. *Australian Veterinary Journal* 89(8), 305–311.

Dyson, S., Berger, J., Ellis, D. and Mullard, J. (2018) Development of an ethogram for a pain scoring system in ridden horses and its application to determine the presence of musculoskeletal pain. *Journal of Veterinary Behavior* 23, 47–57.

Geutjens, C.A., Clayton, H.M. and Kaiser, L.J. (2008) Forces and pressures beneath the saddle during mounting from the ground and from a raised mounting platform. *Veterinary Journal* 175(3), 332–337.

Gunkelman, M., Ryan, F., Keiper, C. and Hammer, C. (2017) Thermography of the equine hoof immediately following trimming and shoeing. *Journal of Equine Veterinary Science* 76, 36–129.

Harvey, A.M., Williams, S.B. and Singer, E.R. (2012) The effect of lateral heel studs on the kinematics of the equine digit while cantering on grass. *Veterinary Journal* 192(2), 217–221.

Hockenhull, J. and Creighton, E. (2012) Equipment and training risk factors associated with ridden behaviour problems in UK leisure horses. *Applied Animal Behaviour Science* 137(1–2), 36–42.

Hockenhull, J. and Creighton, E. (2013) The use of equipment and training practices and the prevalence of owner-reported ridden behaviour problems in UK leisure horses. *Equine Veterinary Journal* 45(1), 15–19.

Jung, A., Jung, H., Choi, Y., Colee, J., Wickens, C. *et al.* (2019) Frequent riding sessions daily elevate stress, blood lactic acid, and heart rate of thoroughbred riding horses. *Journal of Veterinary Behavior* 32, 1–5.

Kydd, E., Padalino, B., Henshall, C. and McGreevy, P. (2017) An analysis of equine round pen training videos posted online: differences between amateur and professional trainers. *PLoS ONE* 12(9), e0184851.

Malone, S.R. and Davies, H.M.S. (2019) Changes in hoof shape during a seven-week period when horses were shod versus barefoot. *Animals (Basel)* 9(12), e1017.

Mansmann, R.A., James, S., Blikslager, A.T. and vom Orde, K. (2010) Long toes in the hind feet and pain in the gluteal region: an observational study of 77 horses. *Journal of Equine Veterinary Science* 30(12), 720–726.

Marsboll, A.F. and Christensen, J.W. (2015) Effects of handling on fear reactions in young Icelandic horses. *Equine Veterinary Journal* 47(5), 615–619.

Moleman, M., van Heel, M.C., van Weeren, P.R. and Back, W. (2006) Hoof growth between two shoeing sessions leads to a substantial increase of the moment about the distal, but not the proximal, interphalangeal joint. *Equine Veterinary Journal* 38(2), 170–174.

Moyer, W. and Anderson, J.P. (1975) Lameness caused by improper shoeing. *Journal of the American Veterinary Medical Association* 166, 47–52.

Murray, R.C., Walters, J.M., Snart, H., Dyson, S.J. and Parkin, T.D. (2010) Identification of risk factors for lameness in dressage horses. *Veterinary Journal* 184(1), 27–36.

Page, B.T. and Hagen, T.L. (2002) Breakover of the hoof and its effect on structures and forces within the foot. *Journal of Equine Veterinary Science* 22(6), 258–264.

Pardoe, C.H., McGuigan, M.P., Rogers, K.M., Rowe, L.L. and Wilson, A.M. (2001) The effect of shoe material on the kinetics and kinematics of foot slip at impact on concrete. *Equine Veterinary Journal Supplement* (33), 70–73.

Proske, D.K., Leatherwood, J.L., Stutts, K.J., Hammer, C.J., Coverdale, J.A. and Anderson, M.J. (2017) Effects of barefoot trimming and shoeing on the joints of the lower forelimb and hoof morphology of mature horses. *Professional Animal Scientist* 33, 483–489.

Scofield, R., Savin, H. and Randle, H. (2013) Road safety: is there a relationship between 'near misses' and the use of rider and horse reflective/fluorescent equipment. In: *Proceedings of the 9th International Equitation Science Conference*, July 17–19 2013, University of Delaware, Newark, p. 30.

Scofield, R.M., Savin, H. and Randle, H. (2014) Riding and road safety: building profiles of leisure riders and their environment in the United Kingdom. In: *Proceedings of the 10th International Equitation Science Conference*, 6–9 August 2014, University of Aarhus, Denmark, p. 41.

Scofield, R.M., Scofield, S.C. and Briggs, E. (2019) Conspicuity equipment and its contribution to the welfare of horse and rider combinations using the road system in the United Kingdom. *Journal of Equine Veterinary Science* 82, e102770.

Scott, E.Y., Woolard, K.D., Finno, C.J. and Murray, J.D. (2018) Cerebellar abiotrophy across domestic species. *Cerebellum* 17(3), 372–379.

Sprick, M., Furst, A., Baschnagel, F., Michel, S., Piskoty, G. *et al.* (2017) The influence of aluminium, steel and polyurethane shoeing systems and of the unshod hoof on the injury risk of a horse kick. An ex-vivo experimental study. *Veterinary and Comparative Orthopaedics and Traumatology* 30(5), 339–345.

Thirkell, J. and Hyland, R. (2017) A preliminary review of equine hoof management and the client-farrier relationship in the United Kingdom. *Journal of Equine Veterinary Science* 59, 88–94.

Thompson, K. and Matthews, C. (2015) Inroads into equestrian safety: rider-reported factors contributing to horse-related accidents and near misses on Australian roads. *Animals (Basel)* 5(3), 592–609.

Thompson, K., McGreevy, P. and McManus, P. (2015) A critical review of horse-related risk: a research agenda for safer mounts, riders and equestrian cultures. *Animals (Basel)* 5(3), 561–575.

Visser, E.K., van Reenen, C.G., Rundgren, M., Zetterqvist, M., Morgan, K. and Blokhuis, H.J. (2003) Responses of horses in behavioural tests correlate with temperament assessed by riders. *Equine Veterinary Journal* 35(2), 176–183.

Visser, E.K., van Reenen, C.G., Blokhuis, M.Z., Morgan, E.K., Hassmen, P. *et al.* (2008) Does horse temperament influence horse-rider cooperation? *Journal of Applied Animal Welfare Science* 11(3), 267–284.

Visser, E.K., Neijenhuis, F., de Graaf-Roelfsema, E., Wesselink, H.G., de Boer, J. *et al.* (2014) Risk factors associated with health disorders in sport and leisure horses in the Netherlands. *Journal of Animal Science* 92(2), 844–855.

von Borstel, U.K., Euent, S., Graf, P., Konig, S. and Gauly, M. (2011) Equine behaviour and heart rate in temperament tests with or without rider or handler. *Physiology and Behaviour* 104(3), 454–463.

Yoshihara, E., Takahashi, T., Otsuka, N., Isayama, T., Tomiyama, T. *et al.* (2010) Heel movement in horses: comparison between glued and nailed horse shoes at different speeds. *Equine Veterinary Journal* 42 (Suppl. 38), 431–435.

Index

Note: The locators in bold and italics represents the tables and figures respectively.

separation anxiety
    appetitive reinforcers 66
    companionship 65
    humane muzzle 67
    laminitis 67
    mitigating factor 65
    pair-bond relationships 65–67, *65, 66*
    perimeter of fence *64*
    social groups 11
shying
    bombproof horse 122
    concerning confidence and riding
        ability 123
    foundation training 121, 122
    hacking on roads *121*
    handlers/riders 121
    horse's stress levels 124
    hyperactive temperament 122
    ultimate resolution 123
    warmblood 124
Skinners box 13, *14*
stabling
    enrichment 8–9
    versus turnout 5–8
standing still
    foundation training 58
    horse pulls and reward of freedom 58
    looping movements 58
    lunge line 59, *60*
    pulling-back behaviour 60
    safety knot, rope 58, *59*
    veterinary surgery 60
stereotypes
    crib-biting 30
    development of 29–30
    locomotory 30

    nursery-type system 31
    oral 30
    prevention 30
straw bedding 9–10, *10*
striking out
    dangerous behavioural repertoire 44, *44*
    dominant behaviour 44
    frustration response 45
    positive reinforcement 45
    punishment 45
    treat-based reward 45

tacking-up
    bridle and bit
        bitless bridles 87–89, 95
        eggbutt snaffle bit 86, *87*
        gag bit *87*
        loose-ring snaffle *86*
        nosebands 88–91
    saddles 91–94
Thorndike's cats *13*
tightness measurement 90, 91
toe calluses *113*
traditionalism 25
training aids 73–76
trial and error learning 13

vascularization 111
veterinary treatment 39

war-bridle 40, 41
weaning 30
willingness 6

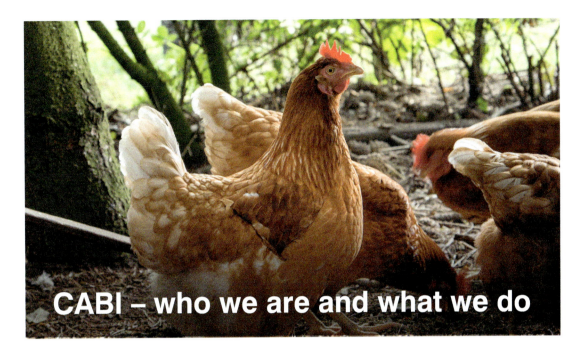

CABI – who we are and what we do

This book is published by **CABI**, an international not-for-profit organisation that improves people's lives worldwide by providing information and applying scientific expertise to solve problems in agriculture and the environment.

CABI is also a global publisher producing key scientific publications, including world renowned databases, as well as compendia, books, ebooks and full text electronic resources. We publish content in a wide range of subject areas including: agriculture and crop science / animal and veterinary sciences / ecology and conservation / environmental science / horticulture and plant sciences / human health, food science and nutrition / international development / leisure and tourism.

The profits from CABI's publishing activities enable us to work with farming communities around the world, supporting them as they battle with poor soil, invasive species and pests and diseases, to improve their livelihoods and help provide food for an ever growing population.

CABI is an international intergovernmental organisation, and we gratefully acknowledge the core financial support from our member countries (and lead agencies) including:

  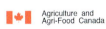

Discover more

To read more about CABI's work, please visit: **www.cabi.org**

Browse our books at: **www.cabi.org/bookshop**,
or explore our online products at: **www.cabi.org/publishing-products**

Interested in writing for CABI? Find our author guidelines here:
www.cabi.org/publishing-products/information-for-authors/